You, Me Conquering Perimenopause & Menopause

How Intermittent Fasting and the Keto Diet Can Help You Get Your Life Back!

Michelle Rowlinson

You, Me Conquering Perimenopause & Menopause
How Intermittent Fasting and the Keto Diet Can Help You Get Your Life Back!
© 2023 Michelle Rowlinson

ISBN: 9798364875228 Paperback

Published by: Inspired Publishing
Cover Designed By: Tanya Grant – The TNG Designs Group Limited

The strategies in this book are presented primarily for enjoyment and educational purposes. Every effort has been made to trace copyright holders and obtain their permission for the use of copyright material.

The information and resources provided in this book are based upon the authors' personal experiences. Any outcome, income statements or other results, are based on the authors' experiences and there is no guarantee that your experience will be the same. There is an inherent risk in any business enterprise or activity and there is no guarantee that you will have similar results as the author as a result of reading this book.

The author reserves the right to make changes and assumes no responsibility or liability whatsoever on behalf of any purchaser or reader of these materials.

Table of Contents

Introduction

I stood in front of my bedroom mirror, crying silently into the sleeve of my dressing gown so that I didn't wake my sleeping son in the next room. The person in the reflection looking back at me was a stranger to me. Who was she? I didn't recognise the tear-stained woman with pain in her eyes. How had I gotten to this point? I didn't even remember becoming her.

She was tired, she was puffy, she was overweight, and she was miserable. Looking at her made me feel beaten.

I had always been a slim girl, naturally sporty with a healthy appetite and a love of cooking. This had always been a winning combination for me, I'd never had to think about my body, except what I would dress it in for my latest night out with my girlfriends.

I'd worked hard to get my pre-pregnancy body back after piling on over four stone with my son, but over the last few years, the weight had started to creep back on to me, no matter what I did. I knew I needed to make some changes. The toll of an unhappy marriage and a son with special needs had made me not prioritise my own needs for a long time.

I tiptoed over the landing and sneaked a peak at my boy. His face was all peaceful in sleep, unlike when he was awake. I felt full of love as I watched him and suddenly decided there and then that I needed to make changes. Big changes!

If I couldn't be strong for myself then how was I going to be strong for him? It was time to take back control! I knew it wouldn't be a case of doing what I'd done before, this time I was going to have to try something new! I'm a determined stubborn woman and I knew that this time I would find the method that worked for me and when I did, I would help other women who had been as desperate as me to get back to their best selves.

Perhaps this all sounds familiar? Perhaps you are struggling with mood swings? Anxiety? Weight gain despite constantly being on a diet?

If any of this rings true to you, then I know you'll have felt my pain and know just what it feels like to be that unhappy. In fact I began writing this book because I never want any woman to feel the way that I did in those dark moments.

My mission in writing this book is for it to help and inform women; women that might be stuck in a cycle of being unhappy and locked in symptoms that they don't understand. If I can help even one woman by sharing my experiences and my knowledge, then I will consider myself successful.

Maybe you feel helpless, trapped in a cycle of restriction then caving in because of how rubbish you feel? Perhaps you have anxiety and panic and feel that nobody understands you and that you're going mad? I'm here to tell you that there IS a way to regain control of your life and your weight to become happy again!

Inside this book are the tools to help you and I am going to walk you through every step of the way.

- We'll learn about what is Perimenopause and menopause and the symptoms you might get
- We'll learn how to manage your mood swings and other perimenopause symptoms
- We will explore the winning combination of intermittent fasting and the keto diet
- I will show you how to begin intermittent fasting safely and effectively
- We will explore which type of intermittent fasting is right for you
- I'll give you tips and tricks to maximise your weight loss

- It will contain delicious recipes to inspire and encourage you on your journey
- We'll learn how to manage the symptoms associated with weight gain
- We'll discuss how to exercise alongside intermittent fasting

So why read my book? What equips me to write a book and tell you what to do?

During my dark times before I found my way through, I have never felt so alone, confused, and miserable. I genuinely couldn't understand what was happening to me. I felt like everything I knew about my body and myself had changed.

It got so bad that I couldn't even go into a supermarket without feeling overwhelmed and anxious. It was only when I fell into a conversation with a colleague at work about menopause that I began to look into potential links with my situation.

Menopause was not something I ever thought about. To me, it was something that happened to older women. My limited knowledge extended to HRT, hot flushes, and an almost jokey narrative of grumpy older ladies.

To my embarrassment it was something I naively thought I didn't need to worry about, especially as a woman in my early 30s.

It isn't a secret that as a society, women's health isn't exactly a priority for discussion, even between women. None of the women in my family or friend circle were different from the average group of women, so it was hardly a surprise that I had never even heard of the term 'peri-menopause'. If only one of them had known half of what I know now!

Trust me when I say I tried them all, every diet under the sun and none of them worked for me, except for this combination of intermittent fasting and a keto-based diet. I can truly say that it changed my life!

Helping women that are in the same place as I was, matters so much to me. I want to share the things that I learnt in this book, because I know firsthand how it feels to be a woman that has lost herself. I lost weight but I also learned about my body and to love it again.

That's how I know that with my help, you can come through what feels like hell and get to the other side.

Would you like to look in that mirror and see the best version of you staring happily in the reflection? Then read on!

Chapter 1

Understanding Your Body Over 40

This chapter is all about understanding the changes that your body will experience as you head towards menopause.

We look in detail at perimenopause and how it connects and intertwines with menopause. We will also look in some detail, at the systems in the body that make menopause happen and what symptoms you might experience during this time.

Menopause is something that we don't tend to talk about until we get to it. When I was growing up it was something that was muttered about behind closed doors. I remember a family friend crassly making a jokey comment about his wife's hot flashes and mood swings. When I asked my Mum about it later on, she shushed me and told me I'd 'understand when I was older.'

As we know, there is a definite reluctance in society to talk about women's health. It may be different for future generations now that we are beginning to live in a more open and tolerant world, but the majority of the people reading this book will have grown up in a world that at best, showed sanitary towel adverts showing blue liquid instead of red and at its worst banned the topic altogether

When I began to experience the symptoms that I now realise were perimenopausal, I had no idea that what was happening to me was hormone based. These are some of the symptoms that I experienced and the way that they manifested in my life.

Weight gain- From the age of 33 I started to notice that my clothes were fitting more tightly than usual. I tried and had mediocre and varied success with countless diets. I even tried the apple diet, eating nothing but apples! I can laugh about it now, but there is part of me that feels sad about how desperate I was. I went from 57kg to 72kg in the space of a year. My son even admitted to me, a year or so later that one of his friends thought that I was pregnant!

Anxiety and depression- The only way to describe how I felt, was crippled with anxiety. There seemed to be no rhyme nor reason to it either. One day I would be on cloud 9 and the next I would be in the depths of despair. In my job as a senior physiotherapist, I managed well to detach myself and put on a professional, happy front. But behind closed doors, it could take the slightest thing to set me off and I would snap at my family and friends for absolutely no reason.

I also experienced panic attacks. I remember one in particular when I was in the cereal aisle at Morrison's. I can laugh about it now, but at the time it seemed like a life-or-death moment trying to decide what sort of cereal I should buy! I felt like my feet were stuck to the floor. I began to cry and started to panic if I was getting the wrong one!

Another time that this panic manifested itself, was when I was driving. I have always been a confident driver, passing my test the first time and I have driven abroad and up and down the country more times than I can remember. However, on one occasion I tried to parallel park downwards on a hill in my car, it wasn't a particularly difficult manoeuvre and one that I'd done a hundred times. On this occasion I went cold, started to hyperventilate, my legs went to jelly, and was completely unable to do it. I eventually managed to pull myself together to get the car in as I was blocking the road, but I had to call my partner to come and move the car out again for me as I was petrified of rolling back into the car behind. I was devastated, I'd always been a strong independent woman. I genuinely at that point thought there was something wrong with me.

Brain fog- I had periods of time where my brain just couldn't concentrate at all. It was like being underwater all of the time. I felt stupid like I'd lost any sort of intelligence. Even small things, such as remembering patients' names, became a major task. I would walk into a room and stand there like an idiot, completely blank. This was particularly scary to me because of my family's history of dementia and Alzheimer's.

Insomnia- I'd suffered from periods of insomnia all my life, which I now realise was a side effect of my endometriosis. However, around my perimenopause, the episodes kicked up a gear. I would lie there for hours on end, and if I was lucky, eventually fall into a patchy disturbed sleep.

Hair loss- I have always had very thick hair, which I was so grateful for as I lost my hair in clumps. I noticed hair all around my house, on the headrest of the car, and stuck to all of the carpets. I remember my vacuum being completely clogged up with hair all wrapped around the brush of it. I had to cut it away with scissors!

Heart palpitations- I experienced heart palpitations, which a doctor diagnosed as part of my anxiety and put me on anti-depressants. These didn't help at all and I continued to have fluttering in my chest, a rapid heartbeat and some chest pain. I got it checked out, as sadly my Father had a heart condition but thankfully I was clear on that front. It later became clear that the heart palpitations were just another symptom of my perimenopause.

Loss of sex drive- I completely lost any sort of sex drive. I had always had a healthy appetite for sex and the fact that it had absolutely disappeared was an extra strain for my husband and me in our marriage. He hadn't done anything wrong, yet the thought of being touched, was more than I could cope with. How do you explain to your partner that the thought of sex repulses you? I had no answers for him or myself

None of these symptoms were in any way helped by the fact I had a lot going on in my personal life, as well as caring for my son who has Aspergers. Eventually, my marriage ended and my personal situation stabilised. I found happiness in a new and loving relationship. But when these physical and mental feelings didn't disappear, I soon realised that there was something else going on, that had nothing to do with my life circumstances.

Let's begin by asking what exactly is perimenopause?

Simply put it is the period of time in a woman's life leading up to menopause when her cycles are no longer predictable. It can last for between four and fifteen years and can begin as early as in a woman's 30s. The symptoms of perimenopause, the age you are when it begins and how long it lasts varies amongst women. According to research by the charity Wellbeing of Women, it is estimated that there are around 13 million people who are currently perimenopausal or menopausal in the UK, this is equivalent to a third of the entire UK female population! **(Source 1)**

This transitional time begins the body's natural progression toward the end of its reproductive years.

So what are the first signs of the perimenopause? Most women find that the first sign is irregular periods. Women will generally go from having a fairly regular menstrual cycle to an unpredictable one.

The main symptoms of perimenopause are the following:

- Hot flashes
- Vaginal dryness
- Anxiety / depression
- Brain fog
- A decrease in memory and concentration
- Loss of sex drive

- Urinary urgency
- Incontinence
- Weight gain
- Mood swings
- Erratic menstrual cycle
- Heavier flow of period
- Hair loss
- Muscle tension/pain
- Insomnia

It is incredible to me that with a third of the females in this country affected by this transitional period in a woman's life, there isn't more being done to support and educate women about what will happen to them.

So what makes the perimenopause begin? In order to understand perimenopause we need to understand what's going on inside our body as it prepares for menopause. This next stage in a woman's life is complicated and scary, but by understanding what's happening inside our incredible bodies, perhaps we can be more prepared.

Let's break it down into sections.

The Endocrine System

The endocrine system is a network of glands and organs located throughout the body. It is similar to the nervous system, in that it regulates the body's functions but whereas the nervous system sends electrical impulse signals from the brain, the endocrine system uses chemical signals called hormones. These hormones travel around the bloodstream to various organs in the body delivering messages and telling them how to function. The endocrine system controls metabolism, sleep cycles, appetite, body temperature and sexual function. The endocrine system is also responsible for reproduction. It sends messages to the ovaries to cause them to produce oestrogen and progesterone. **(Source 2)**

Oestrogen and progesterone are the two hormones that give the body the signals to ovulate and menstruate (releasing eggs and bleeding) As we get older our oestrogen levels start to decrease. This is because the body produces less and less of it as it prepares to stop releasing eggs altogether. As this oestrogen level dips, it affects the progesterone, throwing everything off balance. The majority of symptoms from the menopause are due to declining levels of oestrogen.

- Erratic menstrual cycle- it is the fluctuation of these hormones that cause periods to become irregular and erratic. Eventually, the

14

body makes so little of the oestrogen hormone that the ovaries no longer release eggs and this is what makes the periods stop.

- Light/Heavy flow- the oestrogen levels in our body have an impact on blood flow during menstruation. When there is an excess of oestrogen, it stimulates the uterus to grow a thicker lining, meaning a heavier flow. A heavy flow period means the levels of oestrogen are higher, and vice versa.

- Vaginal dryness- also known as vaginal atrophy. As we age, the walls of the vagina become thinner, due to the declining oestrogen, making it itchy and uncomfortable. This can make sex very uncomfortable too as the dryness leads to tightness too, causing pain during intercourse.

- Weight gain- menopause causes your body to reserve energy more, which means you won't burn calories and fat as easily. This can lead to weight gain. As we know from being women, our appetites are affected by our menstrual cycle before we are perimenopausal! The hunger hormone 'ghrelin' is found to be significantly higher amongst perimenopausal women. Low oestrogen levels in menopause also have an effect on the hormones that control our fullness and appetite, this could lead women to eat more calories without feeling full.

- Hair loss- menopause can affect our hair, causing thinning, breakage and significant hair loss for many women. This is due to low levels of oestrogen, progesterone and a higher level of testosterone.

- Incontinence- the reduction in oestrogen can cause the thinning of the lining of the urethra. The urethra is the tube that urine passes out of the bladder from. The pelvic muscles around it also weaken and cause what is called Stress Incontinence. Coughing, lifting heavy objects, sneezing and even laughing can cause urine leakage. Urine urgency is caused by irritated bladder muscles and can also be an issue in perimenopause. This is when you have a sudden and frequent urge to urinate. This can also result in urine leakage.

The Immune System

As we get older, our immune system declines naturally and doesn't work as well as it did when we were younger. There are many factors that determine how well our immune system works, but the main thing that determines our immunity is a small organ called the Thymus. **(Source 3)**

The Thymus produces cells that in turn become something called T-cells. These t-cells arrange our body's immune response when there are infections.

\

The thymus, shrinks in size as we age, meaning that it produces fewer of the cells that become T-cells. This leaves us more susceptible to disease and inflammation. Men and women alike experience thymus shrinkage, but because of the hormonal changes that women go through in menopause, we tend to have worse effects. The oestrogen and progesterone that our endocrine system makes act as a natural boost and supports our immune function. As we know, when we begin our menopausal time, our oestrogen and progesterone levels are spiking. When those hormones start to spike during the menopause we lose this boost.

There are other symptoms of the menopause that weaken the immune system. As we know insomnia is a common problem for menopausal women. Good quality sleep is essential for keeping a strong immune system.

This lack of sleep can also have a 'knock on' effect. The fatigue experienced from insomnia in turn could affect women's likelihood of exercising or eating a healthy diet. All things that are essential for keeping our immune systems strong.

All of these changes are difficult for women. The many symptoms including weight gain, hot flashes, irregular periods and hair loss can be really stressful. Of course we find ourselves in a vicious cycle by which the stress hormone cortisol is released, which in turn weakens our immune response!

No wonder women struggle to navigate through this minefield of change!

The Nervous System
The first signs we tend to experience of our perimenopause are irregular and erratic periods. It would be fair to assume then, that our menopausal changes begin in our reproductive organs. As we know, our endocrine system controls the hormones that trigger those changes, but the origin of these signals occurs in the brain. The brain and the ovaries are in constant communication, therefore the status of your reproductive system is linked to the health of your brain.

Oestrogen is not only involved in reproduction but in brain function. Therefore during menopause levels decline and affect your brain function, which in turn causes the symptoms of menopause, which are:

- Hot flashes- inside the brain is a structure called the Hypothalamus, which is the link between the endocrine system and the nervous system. Among other things it keeps your body temperature regulated. When the oestrogen doesn't activate the Hypothalamus properly, the brain can't regulate body temperature and that is what causes the hot flashes.
- Insomnia/disturbed sleep- the lack of oestrogen flow also has effects on the brain stem, which plays a role in the REM sleep cycle. Again, it is this drop in oestrogen that doesn't activate the brain correctly, causing disturbed sleep.
- Mood swings/ brain fog- this is down to the amygdala which is the part of the brain that deals with emotions. The ebbing of oestrogen is what makes you experience mood swings and or brain fog.
- Anxiety and depression- the brain is the underlying source of the problems of anxiety and depression during menopause

as the levels of serotonin and dopamine can fluctuate so much during this time.

Dopamine and Serotonin are neurotransmitters, or 'chemical messengers'. These neurotransmitters are used by the nervous system to regulate the processes in your body. Dopamine and Serotonin are widely known as the 'happy hormones', due to their roles in regulating mood and emotion. When released by the brain, dopamine makes us feel pleasure. Serotonin stabilises our moods and makes us feel happy.

These neurotransmitters interact with the oestrogen and the progesterone, which when it fluctuates in menopause, can have a serious effect on these mood-regulating hormones.

As we age, we expect a certain amount of aches and pains. However, at menopause, women's bodies experience a major drop in muscle mass and strength due to that declining oestrogen again! This reduction in oestrogen has an implication on the whole musculoskeletal function, affecting the structure of bone, muscles, tendons and ligaments. A lot of women find that sports they previously excelled in are more painful due to this stress on the body.

- Muscle tension- this is another unpleasant symptom of menopause. Both oestrogen and progesterone have a hand in this! When progesterone is produced, it acts as a muscle relaxant. When these levels decrease during perimenopause muscles become stiff and then contribute to muscle tension.

Oestrogen reduces the collagen content of the tissues in our body, causing increased stiffness in our ligaments and tendons. Oestrogen also helps to regulate the 'stress hormone' called Cortisol. Cortisol rises when our oestrogen levels are too low, causing high blood pressure amongst other things, if this goes on for too long, then the combination of high cortisol and low oestrogen causes the body's muscles to get overtired and tighten.

- Incontinence and urinary urgency- these hormonal changes and muscle tension often impacts our pelvic floor muscles as well. This is a problematic area for lots of women anyway because there is often an underlying weakness from childbirth. This can then have an impact on our pelvic floor muscles leading to decreased bladder control.

What other changes can happen as a result of the menopause?

As if there aren't enough changes to prepare for, there are also indirect changes that may occur when we become menopausal.

- Loss of sex drive- many of the physical changes, experienced during menopause (vaginal dryness for example) can affect your libido. Many women understandably lose their physical confidence when they are suffering from weight gain, hot flashes and urine issues. Not to mention that anxiety and depression are not exactly aphrodisiacs!
- Osteoporosis – this is a condition that affects bone density, making them more fragile. This increases your risk of having bone fractures. Menopausal women are more likely to develop osteoporosis because of the drop in oestrogen levels. Research indicates that approximately 1 in 1o women over 60 years old are affected by osteoporosis worldwide.
- Cardiovascular disease – the oestrogen that we produce offers some protection against coronary artery disease, it helps to control

our cholesterol levels and reduces the risk of fat buildup inside the artery walls. During perimenopause and menopause, the drop in oestrogen increases the risk of the arteries narrowing, as the protective lining caused by oestrogen that used to be there, is no longer as efficient. This increases the risk of developing heart disease or even a stroke. **(Source 4)**

So how do we know when we are out of perimenopause and into full menopause?

Well, as long as you are still having a period, even if it is altered in length or flow, you are still ovulating and therefore still partly fertile. You are considered to be out of perimenopause and into full menopause once you have missed 12 consecutive periods. Most women are into full menopause by the age of 51, but for some women this can be earlier or later.

There are many factors that determine when you'll start your full menopause, including your ovary health, your lifestyle and your genetics. The duration of your menopause can be anything from a few months to ten years, in fact, 1 in 10 women experience menopausal symptoms for ten years following their last period. There is no 'one size fits all' with the length of menopause, just in the same way that no two pregnancies are the same, nor are two menopauses. The same goes for symptoms, some women will have a few symptoms and others will experience most of them.

It is important to remember that although this is a difficult and often upsetting time in a woman's life, it is completely natural. It also won't last forever, even if it feels like it sometimes!

Now, I know at this stage you might be feeling a bit miserable or even want to put the book down. I understand how you're feeling. I've been there! I want you to read on though, while I tell you about another hormone called HGH.

To understand its function let's just revisit what we know about the endocrine system. The endocrine system releases hormones around the body into the bloodstream, sending messages to our organs and telling them how to function.

The human growth hormone (also called HGH) is a hormone released by the pituitary gland. It plays a massive role in body composition, cell repair and metabolism, as well as helping your body recover from injury or disease.

By now we know the effects that oestrogen and progesterone have on our reproductive system and just how much a slight imbalance can have on our entire body.

In adults, the HGH helps to keep our bones and muscles healthy. An adult that has low HGH levels then will suffer from low energy, decreased strength, high cholesterol, and low muscle mass and may also suffer from weight gain due to the fact that our metabolism is also affected by it.

We all know that increased abdominal fat is dangerous to our heart and our risk of cardiovascular disease. There are studies to show that people with higher obesity levels have lower levels of HGH. Therefore losing that abdominal fat will help raise your HGH levels and then improve other areas of your health!

Studies show that dietary fasting leads to a major increase in HGH levels. One study found that 3 days into a fast, HGH levels increased by over 300%. After 1 week of fasting, they had increased by a massive 1,250%

I know from my various attempts at weight loss in the past, that continuous fasting is neither healthy nor sustainable. I knew however, that intermittent fasting worked as I had had some success when I had been on the 5:2 diet (more on that later).

As I learned more about the HGH, I realised that there was a direct correlation with diet. I knew from my previous experience with low carbohydrate diets, that refined carbohydrates and sugar intake are key factors in weight gain and obesity, which also affect HGH levels. **(Source 5)**

I knew then that there must be a way in which to combine intermittent fasting and a low carbohydrate diet, that would not only solve my weight issues but could boost my HGH levels and perhaps help with all of my other perimenopause symptoms!

The next chapters are going to take you through how to start your intermittent fasting journey, how to combine it with the Keto diet for the best results. This is the method that worked for me (believe me, I tried them all!)

Chapter 2

Intermittent Fasting Explained

Intermittent fasting is the practise of eating only within a certain time frame. Intermittent fasting isn't a diet in the traditional sense, in that it doesn't restrict *what* food you eat, but rather *when* you eat it. It is more accurate to describe it as an eating pattern. There is no calorie counting involved on non-fasting days, but it is not sensible to overeat at these times.

The practise of fasting and only eating in at certain times of the day, isn't a new one, it has been done for centuries for health and religious reasons. In fact, fasting was being used as a health aid, as far back as the 5th century when Hippocrates was recommending it to folk for health reasons!

So what happens in our bodies when we practise intermittent fasting?

- Insulin levels decrease **(Source 1)**
  When we eat carbohydrates or sugar, our bodies store any excess that we don't use. When we fast, our blood levels of insulin noticeably drop. This allows fat cells to release any sugar that has been stored, so

that your body can use it for energy, therefore burning fat.

- HGH (human growth hormones) Levels of HGH may increase dramatically **(Source 2)** as we discussed in the previous chapter, HGH has a massive effect on our overall health. Adults that have low levels of HGH suffer from low energy, decreased muscle mass and a decreased metabolism.

One study found that three days into a fast, HGH levels increased by over 300%. After 1 week of fasting, they had increased by a massive 1,250% **(Source 2A)**

- Cellular repair (autophagy)
The body starts important cellular repair processes, such as removing waste material from cells. **(Source 3)** (we will explore this more.)

There are several ways to do intermittent fasting, they all split the time into eating periods and fasting periods. We will go into more detail in the next chapter, but here let's just briefly look at the most popular methods of intermittent fasting:

- The 5:2 diet- with this method, you consume only 500-600 calories on two days of the seven-day week. The two fasting days aren't consecutive. On the remaining five days you eat normally (but not to excess).
- The Eat/Stop/Eat- this involves fasting for 24 hours at a time once or twice a week.
- The 16/8 method- with this method, you restrict your eating to 8 hours of your day only. For example, you could begin your eating period at 1 pm, eat lunch then finish your eating period at 9 pm, having eaten dinner. You would then fast again until the following day at 1 pm, whereby you repeat the process.

The majority of people find the 16/8 method the easiest to stick to. For example, I find that I'm not hungry until lunchtime. My eating window begins at 1 pm when I have lunch. I then eat an evening meal with my family before closing my eating window at 9 pm and then fasting again until the following day.

As women, it's true that we often draw the short straw in the eyes of nature, having to deal with periods, childbirth and the wild roller-coaster of physical and mental change that is menopause. Unfortunately,

Mother Nature doesn't seem to have been any kinder to us about the difference in how our bodies respond to intermittent fasting, compared to our male counterparts!

Let's discuss the different ways that men and women react to intermittent fasting.

Metabolism

Our metabolic response to intermittent fasting is one main difference. Men, as a rule are bigger physically than women and have a bigger body composition. This can be attributed to how we evolved physically through history.

When we lived in a 'hunter-gatherer' society, male and female bodies reacted differently to times of short supply of food. Men's bodies responded to this 'induced fasting' with increased metabolism. This metabolic boost gave their bodies the fuel to be able to hunt when food was in short supply. In contrast to this, women's bodies tend to store and stockpile when their energy supply is threatened, therefore slowing their metabolism down in comparison. (**Source 4**)

Hunger response

When there is a change in the nutrient and calorie consumption in our body, women might react differently to men due to something called Kisspeptin.

In simplistic terms, kisspeptin is a protein-like molecule that has a direct effect on the hormones that regulate hunger, craving and feelings of 'fullness'. Kisspeptin is sensitive to leptin, insulin, and ghrelin, hormones that regulate and react to feelings of hunger and fullness. Our 'hunger hormones' and their release, obviously have an impact on the hunger that we feel.

Women have more kisspeptin than men do, therefore when we fast these levels drop and there may be a shift in our hormone cycle. Compared to our male counterparts, fasting causes women's kisspeptin production to dip.

Insulin and glucose

There aren't lots of studies that compare men and women, with regard to their response to intermittent fasting. However, one of the few studies that does exist, was done on the glucose tolerance of men and women that fasted.

The 2005 study published in 'Obesity Research'(SOURCE 5) tested eight men and women that fasted on alternate days for a period of three weeks. After three weeks the men had experienced improved insulin sensitivity and their glucose response was unchanged.

The women, however, didn't show any change in their insulin sensitivity, but their glucose tolerance was slightly worse than before they fasted.

Another controlled study was conducted with a hundred women that did six months of intermittent fasting. After six months these subjects were found to have decreased insulin levels by 29% and improved their insulin sensitivity.

It's probably safe to say that there isn't enough data to make a full and informed statement on whether men or women have more success at intermittent fasting. However, we know from an evolutionary point of view, that sadly for us women, the composition of men's bodies tends to give them a physical advantage.

The Health Benefits of Intermittent Fasting

As we discussed in the previous chapter, my main desire when I began to research perimenopause and the symptoms I was experiencing, was to lose the weight that I had gained without realising.

While this is of course the main focus of this book, it's important to remember that there are a lot of other health benefits for our body that happen when we fast which have been a vital part of my symptom management as I've navigated through this stage.

Let's explore some of them here.

Cell repair
Autophagy is the body's natural way of regenerating its cells. It's a bit like a cellular spring clean. When nutrients aren't available, damaged and old cells are cleaned out to make room for healthier cells. This involves the cells breaking down and metabolising broken and dysfunctional proteins, that build up inside cells over time.

This increased autophagy has been shown to provide protection against diseases, including cancer and neurodegenerative diseases such as Alzheimer's disease. **(Source 8)** This process triggers a 'clear out' of the old cells in our brain and stimulates new growth, making your brain cells more efficient. This results in better mental clarity and alertness, therefore helping to calm the symptoms of brain fog and confusion that menopausal women experience! **(Source 9)**

Weight loss

When we are fasting, we generally find that our calorie intake is lower as our window for eating is smaller. Obviously, if you are eating to excess during the 'eating' window you will not see the same results. If you stick to the windows of eating and fasting then you will naturally be eating less than you would if you ate from say, 7 am until 9 pm.

The act of eating only during a specific window of time combined with fasting increases our metabolism. Metabolism increases even more with frequent fasting.

A 2018 review of studies in overweight adults found that intermittent fasting led to an average weight loss of 15lbs over the course of 3-12 months. (**Source 10**).

Confidence

The symptoms that have contributed to our mental and physical decline in menopause can absolutely have an effect on our confidence. It doesn't take much to have those feelings of confidence refreshed when we start to see the symptoms that have plagued us, disappear!

As soon as I started to see the weight finally coming off me, after the disappointment and the failure of so many fad diets, it was all I could do not to jump for joy! This feeling then flowed over into other areas of my life and

I began to feel myself again! When I saw other symptoms like my brain fog and hair loss start to stop, I began to lose my anxiety and noticed that my periods of depression were less and less.

Inflammation

We can experience chronic inflammation during menopause which manifests itself in joint pain, asthma, cardiovascular problems, bowel issues, autoimmune diseases and even in cognitive issues like dementia. This is an increasing problem when our oestrogen decline.

A new study has concluded that intermittent fasting reduces inflammation (**Source 11**) The study found that this was in fact due to a reduction in cells that cause inflammation called 'monocytes'.

Heart health

Studies show that intermittent fasting methods can lower blood pressure, blood sugar, and cholesterol, and help with fat and weight loss. Implementing these changes are all ways to improve our chances of avoiding heart attacks, strokes and cardiovascular disease.

HGH (Human Growth Hormone)

When we fast, our HGH levels increase. As we know, the human growth hormone provides us with so many health benefits. Intermittent fasting triggers the production of HGH, allowing fat burning. It enables our body to build muscles, allows fat burning, improves our energy levels and has an anti-ageing effect.

Insulin and glucose
Insulin is a hormone made by the pancreas. This hormone maintains our blood sugar levels and regulates whether our body uses or stores the energy from carbohydrates.

Glucose is a type of sugar that is found in many carbohydrates. When we eat a meal, carbohydrates are broken down and changed into glucose. Glucose comes from the food that we eat and our body's own stored glucose. Insulin then distributes the glucose in our blood into cells all over the body where it absorbs sugar and uses it for energy. If we don't have the right amount of insulin, then glucose can't get into our cells and instead builds up in our blood.

Our body produces a small amount of insulin throughout the day, but the majority of our insulin release occurs when we eat. When we eat, our insulin levels spike. Therefore when we are practising intermittent fasting, we experience fewer of these insulin spikes, firstly, because we are eating less in the first place and secondly because we are eating less often.

When we eat foods that are high in sugar content, such as fruit juices, white bread and white pasta, our pancreas goes into overdrive in producing enough insulin for those levels of blood sugar to be used for energy.

So why do we want to keep our insulin levels down? Well, when our insulin levels are too high the glucose is removed from our blood and is stored as energy. Unless we then use these energy stores, they turn into body fat. Basically, it's impossible to burn fat when we have high levels of insulin in our system.

High increases in insulin not only affect our blood sugar but can also negatively affect cell growth and bodily regeneration. Intermittent fasting not only lowers blood glucose but increases our sensitivity to insulin and reduces inflammation.

The Pros and Cons of Intermittent Fasting

As with everything in life, there are pros and cons. In this sense, the practise of intermittent fasting is no different.

It would be disingenuous to promote intermittent fasting as a 'one size fits all' miracle cure. What will work for one person, won't work for another. Just as one person's menopause isn't the same as another's, not everyone will react or have the exact same results with intermittent fasting.

We will examine the pros and cons of the different versions of intermittent fasting in the next chapters, as well as explore the way the Keto diet works alongside it. We will also be looking at an alternative diet regime in the form of the Mediterranean diet for those that struggle to adapt to the Keto diet.

Whilst we have already explored the various health benefits in this chapter, let's look at a simplified version of the pros and cons of intermittent fasting.

The Pros

Food freedom

Although I found that combination of the keto diet combined with intermittent fasting gave me the absolute best results, I still had measurable success when I was intermittent fasting without a diet plan in place. Granted, my results were better when I combined the two, but I still found that I was losing *some* weight.

If you are someone like I was, that had tried out lots of different fad diets throughout my life; simply limiting the time period that I ate, yet eating my regular diet without strict food limits, felt like absolute food freedom!

Simplification

As any busy Mum will tell you, the daily battle of 'what to cook' can sometimes be overwhelmingly stressful. I found that (especially when I combined intermittent fasting with Keto) the pressure of meal planning was less than before. Once I saw the added benefits of adding Keto into the mix, I found that I enjoyed the boundaries of following food rules, and sticking to time frames. I also enjoyed that there were fewer meals to prepare!

This simplification of 'what and when' when it comes to food, can be a real sustainable lifestyle choice for many.

Mental health benefits

As I said before, there is no magic cure for the symptoms when we enter perimenopause, however, I found that since beginning intermittent fasting, my mental health improved dramatically. I found that my anxiety lessened, my brain fog lifted and my mental clarity improved. This happy change spilt over into the rest of my life improving every aspect of it.

The Cons

Unlearning habits

For most of us we have eaten the same way since we were children. It's hard to unlearn the habits of a lifetime. 'three meals a day' and 'breakfast is the most important meal of the day!' are sayings that have been ingrained into us, societally for many years.

We are creatures of habit, and getting used to changes in our eating and accepting that intermittent fasting requires discipline and planning, may be difficult for some people.

Hunger

At the beginning, you might struggle to adjust to the feeling of hunger. You might even go to bed feeling hungry while your body adjusts to these new feeding patterns. Naturally this is going to feel unpleasant and some people might find this too much to bear. However, our bodies are resilient and adjustable and soon learn new habits. Once you adjust to intermittent fasting, you usually find that you feel less hungry than you used to before. (**Source 12**)

Social life interference/Scheduling

Intermittent fasting can sometimes be hard to schedule, especially if you work shifts, unsociable hours, travel for work or have a busy social life.

However, the beauty of intermittent fasting is that you can make it work for you! Any changes in schedule can usually be accommodated with planning and forethought. If you usually go out for weekend dinners, change them to weekend lunches or vice versa! If you work shift patterns and can't make your two shifts coincide with your eating window? Take the opportunity to do a 24-hour fast for an extra boost and keep things interesting!

Side effects

We will come back to the topic of side effects in a future chapter and look at them in more detail, looking at ways of overcoming potential hurdles and helping you to deal with them.

- Headaches- this is a common side effect when we begin fasting. They usually only last a few days while you adjust to fasting.
- Sleep deprivation- this is usually a result of changes to our eating schedule and for most people settles down after a few days.

- Dehydration/Bad Breath- during the initial days of fasting, the body releases large amounts of salt and water in the urine. If you don't replace fluids and salt, you can become dehydrated. This 'dry mouth' can also lead to bad breath.
- Bloating/Constipation- at the beginning, our digestive system can be shocked by the change to its usual pattern, causing bloating and digestive discomfort. The best way to combat this is to remain hydrated.
- Moodiness- for most people this is just a temporary thing, as we adjust to this new way of life.

For the majority of people, intermittent fasting is safe and simple. As with any major change in our diet or exercise though, we should always consult with a healthcare professional before we embark upon something new.

There is, however, a small section of people that shouldn't practise intermittent fasting and others that should approach it with some caution.

Intermittent fasting is not recommended for the following people:

- Anyone with an eating disorder or a history of eating disorders
- Women that are trying to conceive
- Women that are pregnant or breastfeeding
- Children and young teenagers
- People with immunodeficiencies
- People with dementia
- If you are underweight or malnourished
- Anyone with a history of brain injury or post concussive syndrome

This list is not exhaustive and as I said before, you should ALWAYS check with your healthcare professional before embarking upon intermittent fasting or any new diet.

Chapter 3

Picking Which Type Of Intermittent Fasting Works For You

Picking the right style of intermittent fasting is a very personal thing that depends on trial and error and will be different for everyone.

You might remember I said before that every woman's menopause is as different as every woman's pregnancy. The same principle applies to intermittent fasting. What will work for one will not work for another.

This is why it is so important to try a few methods and not give up if one doesn't work straight away.

Let's dive straight in and look at the different methods and their pros and cons.

The 12:12 Method- Beginner's level
The 12:12 method is probably the simplest of all the intermittent fasting methods. The day is broken down into two sections of twelve hours.

You 'fast' for 12 hours and you 'feast' (feast is a relative term of course!) for 12 hours. This method is also known as 'Overnight fasting' as the fasting window is usually overnight.

For example: If you finish your evening meal at 7 pm then you would fast again until 7 am the following day.

This is a particularly good method for beginners because of its simplicity. The key to beginning these fasting methods is to start slowly and give your body a chance to adapt to the routine. For example, you could even start by doing an eight-hour fast, then slowly increase it an hour a day until you get to a full twelve hours.

A 12-hour fast is already enough for your body to experience a shift in metabolism, utilising stored fats and leading to weight loss.

Pros:
- This method is a good starting point for beginners
- It's a good way of getting used to longer fasts.
- Good for breaking the habit of snacking in the evening
- Your quality of sleep might be better if you aren't sleeping on a full stomach.

Cons:

- It takes about 8-10 hours to get into a 'fasted' state. You won't be burning fat for as long as with other fasts.

This is an example of what your eating schedule might look like on the 12:12 plan

Example Fasting/Eating Schedule
Daily: Eat for 12 hours - 7 am-7 pm / Fast for 12 hours - 7 pm-7 am

7 am- Breakfast
1 pm- Lunch
6 pm- Evening meal ending before your fasting window opens again at 7 pm.

Spontaneous Meal Skipping - Beginner's level
This method is another one that I would recommend for beginners at intermittent fasting. It's perfect for those of us that struggle with the mental idea of 'restricting'. It's also good for those of us with busy, ever-changing schedules. This plan is exactly what it says on the tin. You simply skip a meal if you don't feel hungry, or if you don't have time to eat! This gives us the benefit of a fast but without the mental preparation. You can do them whenever you feel like it!

You can begin them whenever you like and as long as you aren't starving yourself completely, you can do them whenever you want.

For example, many busy mums don't get a chance to have breakfast. They might also then remain busy during the day and not have time for lunch, but then enjoy their evening meal with their family.

Pros:

- Flexibility for people that have busy schedules
- Easy to follow

Cons:

- Easy to break from the plan and stop intermittent fasting altogether
- Not as structured

Example Fasting/Eating Schedule

Daily: Eat according to your wishes/ Fast for 24 hours as and when able to/want to

The 14:10 Method - Beginner's level

With this technique, your fasting window is 14 hours and your eating window is 10 hours. For example, you could eat between 9 am and 7 pm and fast between 7 pm and 9 am. Of course, this can be adjusted, depending on what time you get up.

The 14:10 method is a good choice for people that find the 16:8 method (more on that later) too restrictive. It is a very good starting point for women that are eager to start intermittent fasting, as it eases you into the lifestyle and is easy to build on. 14:10 is effective enough for weight loss but will be easier for somebody that struggles with hunger pangs or finds smaller eating windows too restrictive.

Pros:

- 'Eating window' is more flexible
- Good for people that struggle with hunger pangs
- Good for people beginning intermittent fasting

Cons:

- Easier to overeat with a longer 'eating window'

Example Fasting/Eating Schedule
Daily: Eat for 10 hours - 9 am-7 pm/ Fast for 14 hours - 7 pm-9 am

9 am- Breakfast
2 pm- Lunch
6 pm- Dinner

The 16:8 Method/ Leangains Method - Intermediate level

This method is the most popular of all of the types of intermittent fasting.

Your fasting window is 16 hours and your eating window is 8 hours. For example: if you are the 'breakfast-type', you could start your eating window and 7 am and end it at 3 pm. If you can easily skip breakfast and prefer an evening meal, then you could start your window at 12 pm to incorporate lunch and finish at 8 pm in time for an evening meal.

With my work schedule and family, this is the method I prefer and as I've never been a breakfast person, this works well for me.

The potential problems with this method are the possibility that the smaller window of eating can cause you to feel too restricted and to eat more than you would normally eat to make up for the hours spent fasting. This can lead to digestive problems and unhealthy bingeing.

Pros:

- You can arrange your schedule so that you sleep for the majority of your fasting window

- This method is best for fat burning results

Cons:

- If you are a beginner at intermittent fasting, it can be hard to go 16 hours without food

Example Fasting/Eating Schedule

Daily: Eat for 8 hours -12 pm-8 pm/ Fast for 16 hours - 8 pm-12 pm

12 pm- late breakfast/early lunch
7 pm- dinner

The 5:2 Method- Intermediate level

This method is one of the few methods of intermittent fasting that does actually require some calorie counting.

This plan splits the week into five days of eating normally and two days (non consecutive) that you only consume 500-600 calories. These two days might be a Tuesday and Friday for example. I personally would never recommend doing a 500-calorie day on a weekend. For me, the temptation to 'break' the diet, would be too hard when the rest of the world is enjoying their rest and relaxation time.

This method is also good at teaching us to be mindful of calorie intake on the days when we aren't limiting.

It is important to be careful on fasting days not to do anything overly physical due to the restricted calorie intake.

Many people find that splitting the day up into smaller low-calorie meals works well for them, while others find that fasting during the day and using the entire calorie allowance on an evening meal works better. When I tried this diet, I found that a small afternoon snack, an evening meal and an early night snack were the easiest way to handle it.

Pros:
- Your fasting is only done over two days
- Plan fits easily into a busy social life

Cons:
- The calories on your fasting days are very low
- It involves calorie counting

Example Fasting/Eating Schedule
Eat normally: 5 days a week
2 days a week: (non-consecutive) eat a calorie controlled diet over a 24-hour period

Fasting day:
8 am- 100 calorie breakfast
1 pm- 100 calorie lunch/snack

6 pm- 300 calorie dinner

The Alternate Day Method- Advanced level

The method of alternate day fasting is when you have a 24 hour period of fasting with zero calorie intake, followed by a 12 hour period where you can eat whatever you like. Alternatively, on the fasting day, you can have a small meal of 500 calories if necessary. It depends on our circumstances on the day.

This fasting style is quite like the 5:2 diet in style, whereby you have 'fasting' and 'feasting' days. The only difference here is that instead of doing 2 days of fasting, you do it every other day.

Pros:

- If you feel restricted by fasting every day, it's easier to have off and on days

Cons:

- You won't see results as fast, as you are continually going in and out of a fasting state

Example Fasting/Eating Schedule

Eat normally during a 24-hour window every other day/ Fast for 24 hours on the next day: (a small 500 calorie allowance is allowed as an alternative to full fasting)

Fasting day alternative:

12 pm- 300 calorie lunch

6 pm- 200 calorie dinner

The Eat-Stop-Eat Method/The 24-hour fast-Advanced level

This plan shares similarities with the alternate day method, in that there are 24-hour fasting windows. With this 24-hour fast, you fast from dinner to dinner, lunch to lunch or breakfast to breakfast, meaning that you are basically missing two meals at a time but at the same time, never having a day that is without a meal entirely.

Unlike the alternate day method, this method only requires a 24-hour fast once or twice a week. This method also shares similarities with the 5:2 diet, but unlike the 5:2 diet, you do not consume any food on the fasting days.

Pros:

- This plan is good if you have busy days in your week during which, you know you won't miss food as much

Cons:

- You need to be disciplined to do a full-day fast

- Possibility of overeating when your eating window begins again

Example Fasting/Eating Schedule
Eat normally for 24-hour window every other day / Fast for 24 hours on the next day. A small 500 calorie allowance is allowed as an alternative to full fasting)

Example Fasting/Eating Schedule
Eat normally for 5 days a week / Fast for 24 hour period twice a week

Example fasting window:
Day one: 12 pm-begin your fast
Day two: 12 pm- end your fast

The Crescendo Method- Intermediate level
The crescendo method is the plan that is most highly recommended for women, as it's is a gentle way of easing into intermittent fasting. As we discussed before, women are physically predisposed to find intermittent fasting more challenging. The name 'crescendo fasting' describes the method pretty well. In musical terms, 'crescendo' means a gradual increase in loudness. The fasting windows on the crescendo method are smaller than other methods. You begin with a fast for between twelve and sixteen hours, two or three times a week.

You then gradually increase the amount of fasting that you can handle, hence the crescendo.

Let's say for example you choose a Tuesday and a Friday to have as your fasting days with a 14-hour fasting window. You eat a meal at 9 pm on a Monday and then fast until 11 am on Tuesday. You then will eat normally for the rest of Tuesday and up until Thursday night. You eat at 9 pm Thursday night and then fast until 11 am on Friday and then repeat the cycle.

Pros:

- A good plan to slowly build a tolerance to intermittent fasting

Cons:

- Results will be slower, leading to potential discouragement

Example Fasting/Eating Schedule
Eat normally on non-fasting days/ Fast for 14-hour periods for two days- for example Tuesday and Friday

Example fasting window:
Monday:
9 am- breakfast
2 pm- lunch
9 pm- dinner then begin fast

Tuesday:

11 am- break your fast with breakfast

4 pm- snack

7 pm- dinner

Weds: eat normally

Thurs:

8 am- breakfast

2 pm- lunch

8 pm- eat dinner

9 pm- begin your fast

Friday:

11 am- break your fast with breakfast

The Warrior Method- Expert level

The plan was designed by a soldier called Ori Hefmekler, who transitioned into working in nutrition and exercise after leaving the Israeli special forces. The Warrior method falls under the umbrella term of intermittent fasting, therefore the benefits of intermittent fasting still apply when following this plan. However, there is divided opinion on whether this plan is beneficial, or too restrictive in the long run to make it attainable.

This plan endeavours to copy the eating pattern of 'ancient warriors'. The concept is that they ate very little during the day and feasted at night. This method is one of the most advanced intermittent fasting plans as your fasting window is 20 hours and your eating window is only 4 hours. This method also comes with an advised eating plan that you follow for the first 3 weeks to get used to it. This involves alternating low and high fat and low and high carbohydrate food.

During your fasting window, you are encouraged to eat small amounts of snacks such as hard boiled eggs and small portions of vegetables. Your main meal during your 4-hour eating window is not calorie restricted, you simply eat until you are full.

Certain foods are not recommended on this plan, such as fried foods, processed meats and sugar. However, the plan seems to be more about the time frame in which you can eat, rather than what you eat.

Pros:

- The food you are encouraged to eat is healthy and encourages balanced eating choices
- Weight loss effective

- Although restrictive, it offers the same benefits of any other intermittent fasting method
- No calorie counting

Cons:
- It's highly restrictive
- Can lead to overeating during the small eating window
- Potential to lead to disordered eating
- Little research has been done into the method as a whole
- Hard to sustain
- Risk of malnutrition

Example Fasting/Eating Schedule

Daily: Eat for 4 hours - 3 pm-7 pm / Fast for 20 hours - 7 pm-3 pm

Example fasting window:

8 am- snack of boiled egg

1 pm- snack of a cup of cooked vegetables or a small cup of yoghurt

3 pm-7 pm - evening meal stir fry of chicken and vegetables

As we know, women are predisposed to find intermittent fasting more difficult than men, due to the hormone changes and the fact that men are biologically at an advantage. The best we can do is to be kind to ourselves as we find our way and try and test different plans until we find one that works as not everyone responds to these plans in the same way.

So how do we know which plan will give us the best results? We know that a softer method is better for women to start their fasting journey.

When I began fasting, I went into it headlong. I had made the decision to do it and I was filled with all of this positive energy and resolve! I went straight into a 16/8 fast and was really upset when I crashed a few days later and broke my fast entirely. It's easy to get swept away with enthusiasm especially when you want to see quick results. Take it from me, slow and steady wins the race! It is particularly recommended for women to start slowly so that the body isn't as shocked by the change. Therefore the crescendo, the 12:12 and the 14:10 are the obvious choices to begin with.

Spontaneous meal skipping is also a way to get an idea of how fasting will affect you, but it can be slow to see results which may be disheartening.

Whichever plan you choose, it is still important to eat well during the non-fasting periods. Intermittent fasting can be tricky; it's important to make sure that your body is getting the best nutrition in order to fuel itself for the fasting times ahead. If you eat calorie-dense foods during your eating windows then it's unlikely that you will enjoy the same weight loss and health benefits. I believe that a combination of keto (low carb-high fat) eating and a fasting plan that fits in with *your* lifestyle, is the best way to power your body and see results. As well as the keto diet, I also had success with the Mediterranean diet and intermittent fasting. This is important to mention because, just as all intermittent fasting plans won't suit everyone, neither will all eating plans. We will explore more about these combinations in the following chapters.

As a rule, women are advised to take a gentler approach to fasting than men. Plans with shorter fasting periods and fewer fasting days are recommended. The Alternate day method and the 5:2 allow a small amount of calories, on fasting days are also slightly gentler to follow and having the option of consuming a small number of calories on days that are supposed to be fasted days, such as the alternate day method is best.

Fasting Rules:

- Hydration is key! Drinking water, black coffee and herbal teas can help during those tricky fasting periods but is also essential for keeping us hydrated.

- Listen to your body, if you start to feel really unwell then stop and try again another time or try another method.
- Start small, Rome wasn't built in a day! Don't go straight in for the warrior method if you haven't tried intermittent fasting before.
- Start your plans on days when you know you'll be busy.
- If you fall off the wagon, don't worry! Be kind to yourself and listen to your body. If you beat yourself up about it, you're more likely to give up completely.

Chapter 4

Stages Of Intermittent Fasting

In the previous chapter we discussed the different types of intermittent fasting, the pros and cons of certain methods and the ways in which your body will change as a result. In this chapter we will examine what happens inside your body as you fast, go through the details of each stage in some detail and the effects that they may have and the things you might experience as a result of it.

There are multiple stages of fasting and each stage provides us with different benefits, depending on the length of your fast.

In this chapter, we will look at the main stages of fasting, what happens to our body during these stages and the benefits that come from each stage.

The Fed state (0-8 hours)

Let's first talk about what's called the 'fed state'. This is the time within the first few hours after eating when your body digests the food in your stomach and absorbs the nutrients. The time that it takes to come out of the fed state and into the 'fasting' state, will vary from person to person, as it depends on what food you've eaten and how much you've eaten. At this point, there are changes in certain hormones. There is a decline in the hormone that stimulates hunger, called Ghrelin.**(Source 1)** There is subsequently an increase in Leptin, a hormone that suppresses appetite. **(Source 1.1)**

The human body takes its energy from two sources, the food we eat and stored energy. When we consume food, naturally our body takes its energy from that, rather than the stores of energy that we have in reserve. These reserves are essential as we need to have a continual source of energy to stay alive and keep our organs working.

When we eat, our blood sugar levels increase and insulin is discharged around the body. The amount of insulin released depends on what kind of food we have eaten, how many carbohydrates are in it and how sensitive we are to insulin. It's worth noting, that the highest levels of insulin are released when we eat carbohydrates. We will explore this more in future chapters.

Stage 1: Fasting (8-12 Hours): Stable Blood Sugar
The time that it takes to enter 'fasting mode' varies from person to person, but in general we enter fasting mode between 8-12 hours after our last meal.

As we get into our fast, our glucose (blood sugar) starts to dip. At this point, you might start to feel tired, hungry and irritable. This is the point that a lot of people give up. It can all feel a bit overwhelming. However, after this point, the symptoms start to pass and it becomes easier as your glucose levels stabilise. We discussed this in some detail in Chapter two. **(Source 2)** When we begin fasting, our insulin levels fall and it is this change that signals our body to switch energy sources from food to using glycogen stores from the liver for our energy.

Glycogen is your body's store of sugar, which it will use as a source of fuel when the blood sugar levels are reduced. By the 12-hour point, your body is now tapping into its glycogen. It is this change in insulin levels that alerts our body to go from fat storing to fat burning! Eventually, your blood sugar levels will stabilise. If you are a sufferer of diabetes, then this stage of fasting is particularly beneficial to you, as it will increase your body's insulin sensitivity. **(Source 3)**

At this stage you are beginning to switch to the very early stages of ketosis (more on that later.)

Stage 2: Fasting (12-18 Hours): Ketosis, Fat Burning, and Mental Clarity

This is the stage where the body enters into what is called 'ketosis'. So what does ketosis mean? And how do we get our bodies 'into' ketosis?

First, let us look at ketones. Ketones are energy molecules that are produced by the liver from the breakdown of fats. As we know, the body uses its stores of glycogen for energy first. However, when these stores are empty, the body releases fatty acids from its stores which are taken to the liver and turned into ketones. These ketones are then used as the main energy source. **(Source 4)**

This is when your body is said to be in the metabolic state of ketosis. One of the main symptoms of perimenopause and menopause is weight gain. This stage of fasting is ideal for weight loss, because you don't have any food in your system, therefore you burn through your body fat stores faster. Ketones also are known to suppress your appetite, which should help with any hunger pangs at this stage. This part of fasting also decreases the hormone ghrelin which controls the body's hunger signals. There are a number of ways to get your body into the state of ketosis, one is fasting and the other is a low-carbohydrate diet. The ketogenic (keto) diet is absolutely suited to do alongside intermittent fasting because they complement each other so well and can be done in conjunction with each other.

This is why we will be exploring the diet alongside intermittent fasting, in future chapters.

So how easy is it to get into a state of ketosis? As with the fasting state, a lot depends on the individual in question. The size of your last meal and your diet in general, all affect how fast you enter the state of ketosis.

There are signs to tell you if you have achieved ketosis, you can also do urine and breath tests to see if your body is in the keto state. Some of the signs of the keto state are tiredness, decreased appetite and bad breath. **(Source 5)**

As it takes some time to enter into ketosis, there are some methods of intermittent fasting that may not reach this point as the fasting windows are too small. However, the chances of reaching ketosis faster are greater if you are following a low-carb diet. Again, we will revisit this subject later on!

There are also mental health benefits to be had at this stage as ketosis improves our brain function. Studies have shown **(Source 6)** that ketosis has been proven to help in the prevention of brain issues like Parkinson's and Alzheimer's disease. The production of ketones helps with these diseases because the sufferer can't use enough glycogen to manage perception and cognition. The ketones are an extra source of energy. There is a study that shows how those with Alzheimer's disease have seen improved memory scores when tested after having followed a keto diet. **(Source 7)**

Another benefit at this stage of the fasting programme is a potential boost of something called 'brain-derived neurotrophic factor; or BDNF. BDNF is a protein made in the brain that protects brain cells. BDNF encourages brain health and enhances learning. **(Source 8)**

Stage 3: Fasting (24 hours): Autophagy and Anti-ageing

After the 24-hour stage of fasting, our body begins to start the amazing process of 'autophagy'. We touched on this in a previous chapter but let's look a little more closely at what it means and what happens to your body when it occurs.

The Greek literal translation of autophagy is 'self-eating'. When our bodies are under the 'stress' of a fast, our cells become more efficient. Think of it as a self-preservation system and is the body's way of regenerating its cells. The cells are checked for damaged or dysfunctional parts. They then recycle certain parts, destroy the broken cells and regenerate new and healthy cells.

So what are the benefits of fasting-induced autophagy?

- Brain cell efficiency- The 'clear out' of old cells stimulates new growth, making brain cells more efficient. This also has an effect on our mental health, easing the symptoms of brain fog and improving alertness.
- Increased protection against neurodegenerative diseases- a 2015 study showed that autophagy has been shown to provide protection by removing proteins associated with diseases such as Huntington's, Alzheimer's and Parkinson's.
- Improved immune response- autophagy may remove bacteria, pathogens and viruses that can cause infections, meaning our immune response is improved. **(Source 9)**
- Risk of cancer lowered- research shows that autophagy may help to kill cancer cells. **(Source 10)**
- Anti-ageing- autophagy lessens as we grow older. Fasting is a good way to combat age related health issues.

Stage 4: Fasting (36-48 hours): Growth Hormone and Recovery

At this stage, we are really getting into some serious fasting! This is not for the faint hearted and this kind of fasting should not be undertaken without consulting a healthcare professional first.

However, if you are at this stage of a fast, there are plenty of health benefits that make it worth your while.

We have already talked about HGH (Human growth hormone) in a previous chapter but we can look in more detail now at what HGH is, the benefits it gives us and what happens to our HGH levels when we fast. The human body produces HGH in plentiful supply in our teenage years and then steadily until we hit our 30s. At this point, our levels begin to decline naturally. HGH is made in our pituitary gland, a pea size gland found at the base of our brain. It is responsible for the growth and helps to maintain our tissues, organs and bones.

Let's remind ourselves of the benefits of increased HGH levels:

- increased muscle mass
- muscle repair
- boosts metabolism

- keeps bones healthy

Our pituitary gland makes HGH at the fastest rate when it isn't fed. This production is ramped up when we are asleep and when we are fasting.

There are studies to show that we are already making higher levels of HGH by hour 16 of a fast. **(Source 11)**

This is particularly good news because it means that even if you don't do an advanced method of intermittent fasting like 'warrior' method, you are still benefiting from *some* increase in HGH. However, it does seem that the longer the fast, the better when it comes to HGH levels. A study found that a group of healthy adults that fasted for 48 hours showed a 400% increase in HGH. **(Source 12)**

Below is a table of guidelines for predicted HGH increase at different fasting times. However, these are estimates, everybody's HGH levels are different and this is just for guidance.

Fasting Period	Human Growth Hormone Increase
8 Hours	100%
16 Hours	200 – 300%
24 Hours	400 – 500%

36 Hours	700 – 800%
2 Days	1000%
5 Days	1250% +

We know that fasting increases our HGH levels in itself. We also know that the pituitary gland makes more HGH when we are asleep. Therefore, for an extra boost, it makes sense to try and elevate our levels even further by shifting our fasting window so that we are in our fasted state earlier in the day. For example, assuming you are following the 16/8 method, you could set your eating window from 9 am to 5 pm so that once you go to bed, you are further along in your fasting state.

Stage 5: Fasting (72+ hours): Stem Cells and Immune Function

A 72-hour fast is not one to undertake lightly and as previously stated, this should be done with care and under the guidance of a healthcare professional. However, there are further benefits to be found by doing a fast for as long as this.

- Cell regeneration- At this stage in fasting, stem cell regeneration takes place. A 2014 study showed that a fast for 72 hours caused an almost full rejuvenation, breaking down old immune cells and making brand cells in place of the old ones. **(Source 13)** This means the immune system has had a near complete overhaul.

- The same study mentioned above, also studied the effects of cancer patients that fasted throughout chemotherapy. Despite its obvious benefits to cancer patients, chemotherapy is a double edged sword, in that it also negatively affects the immune system, leaving patients at an increased risk of infection. This study showed that when patients fasted prior to their chemo sessions, it mitigated some of the negative effects of chemotherapy. **(Source 14)**
- Continued autophagy / fat burning- all of the benefits that are found at earlier stages of fasting have now increased in their strength.
- Deeper ketosis- after 72 hours of fasting your body is now running solely on stored fat, this will be initiating weight loss.

It's important to be careful when ending a long fast, the digestive system is effectively hibernating after a long fast and it shouldn't be shocked by dealing with too much food at once. Eating too much food at once might cause you to experience nausea, diarrhoea or stomach pain.

- Keep drinking- It's essential to remain hydrated at all times during a fast, but keep up the liquid intake when leaving a fast. Water is best of course but herbal teas, clear soup and broth are gentle too.
- Introduce food slowly and in small amounts.
- Stick to low carb and high fat meals.
- Don't eat anything too processed or sugary to avoid insulin surges.
- Give yourself two days to ease back into eating normally.

Chapter 5

Secrets Tips On How To Overcome Obstacles And Maintain Intermittent Fasting

It's easy to get overwhelmed by the idea of intermittent fasting. In the western world we are conditioned by tropes such as 'three meals a day" and "breakfast is the most important meal of the day". From a societal point of view, fasting is not generally seen as acceptable. There are a lot of people that have a lot of strong opinions about whether fasting is 'safe'. Things are changing however with the surge of diets like the 5:2 coming into popularity over the last 10 years. However, there is still a lot of misinformation out there, both positive and negative.

Intermittent fasting won't be for everyone, as we know. There are people that aren't advised to fast due to varied reasons such as medical conditions and age. There are other folks, like me that consider intermittent fasting as the saviour of not only their physical health symptoms but their mental health too.

Intermittent fasting is more of a lifestyle, it's never going to be perfect because we aren't perfect as human beings. We will have good days and bad days and that's ok.

One of the first things that changed for me when I was finally successful at reaching my weight loss goals, was my feelings about my own body. For the first time in my adult life, I approached my body and myself with kindness. I grew up in the 90s when diet culture was at its most toxic. I read the magazines with the 'circle of shame' around pictures of celebrities. I felt pressured to embrace the look of 'rail thin' and 'heroin chic'. We were taught negativity about our bodies and I, like many women my age, struggled to appreciate my body for the incredible thing that it is, despite its perceived imperfections.

It's important to remember that your body is the only one you'll ever have, you need to treat it with respect and love.

To begin your intermittent fasting journey from a place of kindness to yourself will make the experience far easier and far more productive.

It's helpful to find your motivation, having a clear sense of your goals and what you want to achieve will help you to get the end results you desire. Try and imagine how you'll feel when you start to see results, when you see your body changing and your symptoms easing. Hold that picture in your mind when you have wobbles, (because you will have wobbles, that's inevitable!) and use it as your motivation to get back on to it.

I know how disappointing it feels when you 'fall off the wagon' with a diet plan. I've done it plenty of times, you slip and then you think 'well I've ruined it now'. That then causes a spiral and most people then give up. Whereas if they had just accepted the wobble, acknowledged it and then moved on, the damage would have been much more limited!

You've seen the evidence that fasting works, there's no reason why it can't work for you. There's no doubt in my mind that a positive mindset has a lot to do with your success at intermittent fasting, but let's talk about some other tips that might help you on your journey.

- Go gently- Don't get ahead of yourself. Choose an intermittent fasting plan that's not too hardcore and don't be afraid to change it if it isn't working for you, or if you find it too hard. It's a marathon, not a sprint!
- Get organised- Getting in control feels good! Make sure you do a meal plan for your first

week or so. The last thing you want is to get to your eating window and have nothing in the fridge or not know what you're having to eat. You'll find that you'll be more likely to sway from your eating plan if you aren't organised.

- Keep hydrated- We will talk later on about food tips and what to eat, depending on what food plan you're following. Hydration is really important to your body at all times especially when you're fasting.

- Get enough sleep- Not only is sleep a good way to spend a good chunk of your fasting hours but getting enough rest is beneficial. When we don't sleep our cortisol (stress hormone) levels rise. High cortisol levels have an impact on your insulin levels too and can increase sugar cravings and comfort foods.

- Listen to your body- Recognise when you need to take a break from fasting. We know that fasting is generally harder for women, so allow yourself moments of respite if you need them.

- Be mindful of food- We know that the focus of intermittent fasting is on when you eat, rather than what. However, it isn't going to help with your weight loss or general health if you use your eating windows poorly. It's easier than you think to eat a day's worth (or more!) calories in one eating window. Make sure your meals are filling, balanced and full of nutrients.

The subject of hunger is one that will affect us all differently. We will all experience hunger in various ways, depending on our schedules, our hormones and our lifestyle. It's helpful to think about the distinction between hunger and appetite. It's a given that we will all feel hungry when fasting. The key is learning to honour that feeling, recognise it and separate it from our brain's desire to eat from an emotional need or as part of a pattern that we've followed for years.

While we are on the subject of food, let's look at some specific tips on how to handle hunger cravings.

- Eat more protein- Make sure you are eating enough protein during your eating windows. When we eat meals that are high in protein, the body's ghrelin (hunger hormone) decreases.
- Keep busy- Many people eat out of boredom. I was the worst offender for this! Finding a

hobby or focusing on work can really help in more difficult moments of fasting.

- Drink coffee and tea- As long as you're keeping your drinks calorie free when you're fasting, having some interesting drinks helps with hunger pangs. They can also decrease your feelings of hunger. Alternatively, you can drink carbonated water for a taste of something fizzy.

- Avoid alcohol- Alcohol causes insulin spikes and more often than not, leads to 'alcohol munchies' after a few too many! Not to mention hangover cravings. Of course, there are going to be times in your life when you want to have drinks. It's a natural part of life and one that you shouldn't deny yourself. Try and stick to low carb drinks to limit any damage, such as champagne, dry wines and pure spirits with 0 sugar/carb mixers.

The transition from your old eating habits to your new intermittent fasting plan can be a tricky one. There are changes and side effects that you might experience as you navigate your way through.

Digestive issues

As your body adjusts to the change in your eating habits and the difference in eating schedules, you might find that you experience side effects in your digestion.

Constipation is a common side effect, it happens for a couple of reasons. Firstly, because we aren't drinking enough water and our body becomes dehydrated. Secondly, when we fast there will be less 'matter' to pass through our bowels to make stools. The softness of your stools will depend on what food is being eaten. If you are following a low-carb diet such as the keto diet then you will find that it's easy to end up not eating enough fibre. Fibre is essential for keeping the bowel moving. To combat this, it's important to drink between 6-8 glasses of water a day and to make sure the meals you eat during your eating window are balanced in nutrients. If you are on the keto diet, there are plenty of fibre-rich foods you can eat without getting out of ketosis, such as avocado, nuts and green vegetables. (More on this later.)

Another digestive issue, but at the opposite end of the scale is diarrhoea. There are a couple of reasons why this might happen. It's fairly rare to have diarrhoea when you are in your fasting window, it usually occurs once you start eating again. Your digestive system slows when you aren't eating. If you then start eating again with a big meal then this can shock your digestive system and make it hard for it to digest. Excess caffeine can also give you diarrhoea. A lot of people rely on coffee especially to help them through their fasting windows, but if you suffer from diarrhoea then it might be best to leave it out of your diet.

Another reason for diarrhoea is an excess of electrolytes. People that are fasting often supplement their diets with electrolytes such as magnesium and sodium to prevent dehydration. An excess of electrolytes can cause diarrhoea. **(Source 1)**

It's common to experience nausea when you're fasting. Your stomach is used to a routine of digesting food at a certain time (usually three meals a day). During digestion, food comes into the stomach to be broken down by an acid called Hydrochloric acid. This acid keeps being released as normal (while your body adjusts to new feeding times). This excess of acid can lead to nausea.

This symptom should ease up, once your body gets used to your new fasting routine. You can also suffer from bloating when you begin fasting. It is generally caused by dehydration, digestive changes in routine and a lack of fibre, much like the other symptoms. Although it can be painful and upsetting to suffer from side effects like these, the good news is that most of them settle down after a few days.

Here are some tips for relieving nausea and bloating:

- Peppermint tea- Peppermint is well known for relieving nausea and can be taken in tea or capsule form.
- Ginger- Chewing on ginger root, sipping ginger tea or taking ginger capsules can all alleviate symptoms of nausea and bloat.
- Take a walk- Gentle exercise and fresh air can do wonders for ridding yourself of nausea
- Yoga- A gentle run through of some simple yoga poses, including 'happy baby', 'child's pose' and even lying flat can be helpful to your mind as well as digestive issues
- Don't over-eat- the temptation to stuff yourself can be overwhelming when you are hungry from a fast. Try to eat a small portion first, especially after a long fast, then wait twenty minutes and see if you are still hungry before eating more.

Irritability and mood changes

It's quite normal to become irritable when we feel 'deprived' of food, especially if we are used to eating as and when we feel like it. A restriction in food can also cause a release of the stress hormone cortisol, leading to irritability and grumpiness. Another reason for irritability may be the change in blood sugar when we fast. Low blood sugar has been linked to irritability and moodiness. **(Source 2)** The good news is that these effects are temporary as your body gets used to its new regime.

It's important to remember that while there are physical reasons for moodiness and irritability when fasting, there is a good chance that these symptoms originate from a place of emotion too.

Many of us have been raised with the idea of food as a reward or a recompense. Had a bad day? Have something sweet to make you feel better. Had a bad breakup? Eat a whole chocolate cake to get over it. Food is ceremonial, it's celebrational, we do eat when we are sad and when we are happy! This is not a book that demonises emotional eating, there is a societal need to share food with our loved ones, to cook for each other and to celebrate. To deny that would be out of touch. However, there is a need to identify true hunger and acknowledge the difference between that and irritability because we feel deprived of our favourite sugary treat. A lot of irritability will subside when you begin to reap the benefits of intermittent fasting, leading to a happier relationship with your body and hopefully your mind.

Fatigue and low energy
Feeling more tired and lacking in energy are fairly common side effects of fasting. This can be for a variety of reasons, or a combination of some.

- Dehydration- There is evidence that when you become dehydrated, your blood pressure drops. This can lead to a reduction in the flow of blood to your brain. This makes you feel sleepy and lethargic. Try to keep up your fluid intake to avoid this.
- Poor diet- Make sure you are eating a balanced diet, avoiding processed food and sugars.
- Check your calories- Ensure you are eating enough! Depending on the fasting method and your lifestyle, there's a possibility you might not be consuming enough calories. Remember, your body needs calories for energy.

Sleep disturbances

You have probably heard of something called Circadian rhythms. This is basically our body's internal clock. When you're restricting your eating window with intermittent fasting, your circadian rhythms have been altered.

Your body will take a little time to get used to the change in eating habits, but after a few weeks, you will feel better. Another reason for the lack of decent sleep is due to the rise in cortisol and insulin in our bodies when we are fasting. REM or 'Rapid Eye Movement' sleep, is especially important to our bodies because it is the section of the sleep process that is key to keeping our central nervous system functioning properly. One study discovered that it could be this rise in these hormones that decrease the amount of REM sleep that the body gets. **(Source 3)**

Another thing to remember is, that if your eating window ends a long time before your bedtime, then it can be grating to go to bed with a grumbling tummy. This is one of the reasons why I have always found that scheduling my meals so I start my eating window later in the day, works best for me.

So how can we combat sleep disturbances?

- Avoid caffeine- Caffeine is a stimulant. Try and avoid it from early evening and stick to herbal teas and cold drinks.

- Avoid alcohol- Alcohol might make you go to sleep quicker but it disrupts the REM sleep cycle and decreases sleep quality. It can also cause broken sleep.

- Increase your protein- There are studies to show that meals that are high in protein, decrease ghrelin. (the hunger hormone). Ghrelin is also responsible for increasing our metabolic rate when we sleep. **(Source 4)**

Bad breath

An unfortunate side effect of fasting is unpleasant breath. When you are fasting and have an empty stomach for a long time, there can be a stale smell. Most of us have experienced a nasty taste in our mouths when we've had prolonged gaps between meals, this is an extension of that. When our stomach doesn't receive food when it expects, the release of digestive fluids reacts with the stomach lining, which can release an unpleasant smell.

If you are doing the keto diet alongside fasting then there is also the issue of keto breath. Keto breath is caused by the excess of ketones leaving the body when your body is in ketosis. It can smell fruity and acidic. It's harmless and in some ways, it's a good thing as it tells you that your body is now in ketosis and burning through your fat stores. However, aesthetically it's not very pleasing.

Try these tips to lessen the bad breath:

- Drink lemon water- Not only will staying hydrated help your overall health when fasting, but lemons have antibacterial properties that kill off bacteria lurking in your mouth.
- Chew on mint leaves- It might sound a bit far out, but chewing on fresh herbs is a better alternative than eating breath mints. These often have hidden sugars, which can kick you out of ketosis.
- Dental hygiene- Although keto breath and fasting breath will occur regardless of hygiene levels, it can't hurt to give yourself an extra oral hygiene boost! Flossing in particular gets rid of any lingering pieces of food that can get stuck between teeth and begin to smell.

Dehydration

Most of the side effects we have discussed in this chapter have roots in dehydration. Our bodies require lots of water when we fast for a couple of reasons. Firstly, when we begin fasting, the body releases large amounts of water and salt in our urine.**(Source 5)** If you don't drink enough fluids to replace this water and electrolytes then you can become dehydrated. Secondly, the human body needs extra hydration when you fast, because low levels of insulin, which we have when we fast, lead to dehydration.

Keeping properly hydrated solves all sorts of side effects of fasting; try to drink at least 6-8 glasses of water a day.

Malnutrition

Although it sounds dramatic to talk in terms of malnutrition, it is actually a very common and real problem with modern diets. When we picture malnourishment, we usually think of it in terms of being starved or underweight. However, to be malnourished is simply to have an imbalance in the nutrients that your body needs and the nutrients that it has. You can even be malnourished from a vitamin deficiency. Malnourishment is a very real possibility when fasting, especially if you fast over a long period. To avoid this, you need to make sure that you plan your diet so that all of your calorie and nutrient needs are met.

What you can eat and drink during fasting
This may seem like a strange question. Surely if you're fasting, you're not eating anything? While it's true that a true fast would absolutely prohibit any food at all, there are a few exceptions to the rule that may ease you into the practise of fasting. Some studies say that if you keep your carbohydrate intake below 50 grams a day, then you can keep the benefits of the fast and not be 'kicked out' of ketosis.**(Source 6)** However, you must remember that drinking or eating anything with calories, will technically break your fasting period.

Food you can eat while fasting:

- bone broth or clear vegetable broth
- pickle juice
- 50 cal high fat snack (more on this later)

The following is a list of drinks that you can drink freely from, that won't break your fasting:

- unsweetened sparkling water
- black coffee
- black tea

- herbal teas
- water

Supplements

We have already talked about how some people add electrolytes to their diet during fasting, to lessen the chances of dehydration. Others also take dietary supplements to ensure that they are not missing out on any nutrients while they undertake intermittent fasting.

When you are only eating for a short amount of time each day, it is easy to have a diet that is deficient in certain vitamins.

If you do decide to introduce supplements to your regime, it's important to know which ones include sugar or calories and will break your fast and which ones won't.

These supplements are less likely to break a fast:

- Fish oil- These are calorie free and carb-free
- Multivitamins- As long as they are sugar free they should be zero calorie
- Individual supplements- Such as potassium, vitamin D and B (Vitamin A,

D, E and K are better taken with food, so save those for your eating window!)

- Probiotics and prebiotics- As long as they are sugar free!
- Creatine- this is used for athletic performance
- Collagen

These supplements are likely to break your fast:

- Protein powders- These contain calories and will trigger an insulin response, preventing fasting. **(Source 7)**
- Multivitamins in gummy form- These generally contain sugars and fats.
- Sugars- Supplements that contain the words, pectin, maltodextrin, fructose or fruit juice are packed with sugar and calories.

Chapter 6

Foods And Diets That Do And Don't Do Well With Intermittent Fasting

There was a time when I would stand in front of the mirror crying on a daily basis. The unhappy state of my life and the onset of what I didn't realise were perimenopause symptoms, had really taken its toll on my mental and physical health. Once I discovered the combination of following the 16/8 intermittent fasting method alongside the keto diet, I knew that I wanted to share my findings with other women that felt the same way I had.

I found over the time that I had been fasting, that although I had some success following a 'regular' diet with intermittent fasting, it was when I followed the keto diet alongside it, that I really noticed major results. Not only was the weight flying off me, but the symptoms of perimenopause that I'd been suffering from, had really eased. As soon as I tried the keto diet alongside fasting, it was as if everything fell into place. I remember that the first week I lost 5lbs without even noticing. Within a month of fasting alongside the keto diet, my skin had cleared up, I had lost over 12lbs, my hair loss seemed to have halted and my episodes of anxiety had nearly stopped. I found that a low carb diet really suited me and my taste buds.

I had tried the Mediterranean diet too, not long before, which focuses on plenty of vegetables, lean protein and a higher level of carbs. I had some success with this too, although I found that the keto diet just suited me better.

It's worth noting that people's bodies respond differently to certain diets. A good friend of mine tried the keto diet and lost 2lbs in a month, then tried the Mediterranean diet and lost 6lbs in her first week.

In this chapter, we will talk about the benefits of both the keto and the Mediterranean diet when combined with fasting. We will also look at what foods you can eat during fasting (we have touched on this in the previous chapter) and what foods are good to eat when you're outside the fasting window.

First of all, let's focus on the food and drink that you can eat when you're fasting. As we know, eating anything with a calorific value *technically* breaks a fast, however, there are studies that say that if you keep your calories low and the carbs below 50g, then you won't kick your body out of ketosis by having a snack. If you are following the 'Warrior' method, snacks of around 50 calories are built into a version of this plan as a way of building up to a 20-hour fasting window. However, if you can stick to no food during this time then you will reap more benefits.

Let's look at some foods that you can eat that shouldn't kick you out of ketosis:

- Bone broth- This is a clear soup made from stock made by boiling up animal bones. This sounds less than appetising in theory, but it has many nutritional benefits and is rich in vitamins and minerals.
- Healthy fat- A small amount of a high quality healthy fat is ok to have as a snack if you really need it. As long as it's no more than 50 calories worth. A measure of nuts or olives is a good example of a suitable snack.
- Vegetable broth- This is a good alternative to bone broth. As long as the vegetables used are low carb and your calories are low-calorie.
- Gherkin/Pickles and juice- This might seem like an odd one but they contain lots of electrolytes and as long as you are having one of the no-sugar varieties, these are a good savoury option for a snack.

What to drink?

- Coffee- Many of us are reliant on caffeine to get us through the day. Luckily for those of us doing the keto diet, there are now studies to show that coffee increases our ketone production! **(Source 1)** For best results, it is best to stick to black coffee. As an alternative, you can have a small amount of almond milk, as long as it's a sugar free, unsweetened variety with low carb content. As a UK resident, the only one I have found that is suitable and doesn't curdle is the Alpro Almond milk. (not the barista variety!) Adding cinnamon or nutmeg is another good way of jazzing up a coffee.

- Sweeteners- If you usually take sugar in your hot drink, then zero sweeteners such as Erythritol or Stevia are a nice alternative that won't break your fast. Anything with high sugar content such as honey will break your fast and kick you out of ketosis.

- Teas- The same rules apply, avoid milk and sugar and opt for black tea or herbal teas. Green tea, lemon and ginger and peppermint are all flavourful teas to have plain. You can enjoy them iced or hot.

- Apple cider vinegar
- Water- Still or sparkling, just make sure that you avoid flavoured sparkling water. Add lemon, lime or cucumber to water to jazz it up if you want a hint of flavour.

What about diet fizzy drinks? Although technically they are low calorie and low in sugar, many varieties will still break your fast because of the artificial sweeteners they contain. These can have an effect on your insulin levels. In my opinion, it's best to try and make do without them.

When you follow intermittent fasting and arrive at your eating window, technically you are allowed to eat what you like. I followed the 5:2 diet briefly and ate in my normal way on the five normal days. I did have some success with weight loss, but it wasn't until I did the keto combined with 16/8 that I saw major results. The 'freedom' of the 5:2 diet didn't give me enough structure and although I stuck to the fasting days and the low calories, I didn't feel any major health benefits. I also found that I was tempted to really go to town on food on my eating days, as I'd been so hungry on the fasting days. Many people find that this can lead to an excess of calories that really becomes counterproductive to the whole fasting program.

It's important to make sure that our bodies are getting the nutrients that they need as our windows of eating are smaller when we are fasting. We should make sure that our diets are balanced and fulfilling.

Let's look at some examples of foods that are particularly recommended when you're following intermittent fasting without following a particular diet plan but want to have a nutritious and balanced diet.

Avocados

Avocados have experienced a resurgence in popularity over the last ten years after the low fat diets of the 80s and 90s demonised them for their high fat content. They contain what are known as 'healthy fats' aka monounsaturated fat. Monounsaturated fats are the kind of fats that are found in olive oil, olives, eggs and some nuts. Not only are they high in fat, they are also packed with vitamins, fibre and minerals. The fat and fibre content of avocados means that they will keep you fuller, for longer. This is a great reason to add them to your menu when following a fasting program.

Fish

It's highly recommended that we eat at least 2 portions of fish a week. Fishes with the highest fat content are considered to be the most beneficial to our health. Fatty fish like salmon, mackerel and sardines are packed with protein, vitamins, minerals and omega-3 fatty acids. Omega 3 is necessary for brain function, heart health and regulating blood pressure. (**Source 4,5,6**)

Protein
High quality protein is essential while you're doing a fasting program. Studies have shown that it helps you to feel more full. (**Source 2**) It's also responsible for increasing your muscle mass and strength, and for keeping your bones healthy. This is especially important for women that are perimenopausal or menopausal, as we are more at risk of osteoporosis. (**Source 3**)

Some particularly good sources of protein are:

- Beef
- Poultry such as chicken, turkey and duck
- Pork
- Eggs
- Spinach
- Mushrooms

Cruciferous Vegetables
These are vegetables from the cabbage family. They include:

- Broccoli

- Cauliflower
- Kale
- Cabbage
- Turnip
- Brussels Sprouts

They are really high in vitamins A, C and K as well as being rich in minerals and high in fibre. As we know, fibre is necessary for keeping our digestive system working properly. It's important to eat the recommended amount of fibre while fasting. A simple small serving of broccoli can provide us with 3-5 grams of fibre.

Whole grains
Whole grains are basically grains such as rice, oat and barley that haven't been through a processing stage to remove parts of the grain. Whole grains such as barley, oats, quinoa and wild rice are unprocessed and have a better nutritional value than processed grains such as white rice, pasta and white bread. Whole grains provide us with lots of fibre, vitamin B and plenty of minerals.
Try incorporating foods from this list into your eating plan to keep balanced when fasting. Just watch out for hidden sugars in some products such as wholewheat crackers.

- Brown/Wild rice
- Quinoa
- Oats
- Buckwheat
- Wholewheat

Berries

Berries are an excellent source of Vitamin C. Vitamin C is essential in maintaining healthy bones, skin and cells. **(Source 7)**

- Strawberries
- Blueberries
- Raspberries
- Blackberries

The Keto diet

I've mentioned the keto diet in previous chapters and how well it works for me, not just for weight loss, but for easing other menopause symptoms that I experienced.

Let's dive into what the keto diet is and how it works.

First, let's refresh our memories and revisit what ketosis is. As we know, the body uses its stores of glycogen as a primary source of energy. When its glycogen stores are empty, the body takes its energy from ketones, which are produced in the liver from the fat in our food and the fat stored in our bodies. When your body is running from ketones, not glycogen, your body is said to be in the state of 'ketosis'. You can get your body into ketosis by fasting, or by changing your diet.

The idea of the keto diet is to severely limit the body's intake of carbohydrates. When we eat carbs, the body converts them straight into glucose and therefore to glycogen. If we cut our intake of carbs, then our body has to revert to its fat stores for energy, which are then taken to the liver and turned into ketones. These are in turn, used as our main energy source. This process is sped up, if we don't have any glycogen stores to burn through in the first place, therefore putting us into a state of ketosis sooner.

So how is the keto diet constructed? The keto diet is a low carbohydrate and high fat diet. The majority of your calories will come from fat, with some protein and a very small amount of carbohydrates.

A traditional keto diet would be made up of 70% fat, 25 % protein and just 5% of carbohydrates. However, this depends on your individual needs and your own macronutrient needs.

Macronutrients

Let's get straight onto the topic of macros. Macros are short for macronutrients. The calories that you eat, all come from one of the three macronutrients. These are the protein, carbohydrates and fat that food is made of that give us energy. You might have heard about people 'counting their macros'. All that means is that you are counting the grams of protein, carbs and fat that you're eating. It's important to understand that protein, carbs and fat don't all contain the same amount of calories.

- Carbs- 4 calories per gram
- Protein- 4 calories per gram
- Fat- 9 calories per gram

Macro counting is a way of tracking where your calories come from the food that you eat and how they affect your body.

Let's look at an example. The recommended calorie intake for a woman in the U.K is 2,000 calories per day. If you eat 200g of carbohydrates at 4 calories per gram, that would mean that you're eating 800 calories from carbs leaving you with 1,200 calories left to share between your protein and your fat intake.

When following the keto diet, our ratios have to be different to put our bodies into ketosis. If you embark upon the keto diet, you have to split your macros into different ratios, usually approximately 55-60 % fat, 30-35% protein and 5-10% carbs.

Counting macros is a good way of keeping an eye on the exact nutrition that we are getting, especially when we are fasting and following a specific diet, like the keto diet.

Different fats
Not all fats are created equally! Let's take a look at the different types of fat, what they do and where they are found.

- Trans fats- These are chemically altered vegetable oils that remain solid at room temperature. They are found in margarine, vegetable shortening, microwave popcorn and fried foods such as doughnuts, fries and cakes. These are deemed to be the unhealthiest types of fats. They have been linked to an increase of inflammation in the body, putting us at higher risk of heart disease and strokes.

- Saturated fats- These are found in most high fat meats and dairy products such as pork, lamb, chicken, butter, whole milk and cheese. For many years these sorts of fats have been demonised, considered unhealthy and linked to high cholesterol and heart disease. However, in recent years especially with the surge of low carb, high fat diets, this idea has been called into question. **(Source 7b)**
- Monounsaturated fats- These oils are found in nuts, olive oil and avocados. These fats are considered healthy fats and can improve your cholesterol and lower the risk of cardiovascular issues. **(Source 7a)**
- Polyunsaturated fats- Also considered a healthy fat, these are found in fatty fish, seeds, nuts and oils. Polyunsaturated fats supply omega 3 and omega 6 which the body doesn't make, therefore we need to get them from our food. These are essential for our brain function and cell growth. **(Source 7c)**

What to eat

In the next chapter we will look at the food that you can eat on keto and will list specific recipes, looking at everything from breakfasts to snacks and side dishes.

When I first started doing the keto diet, I was excited to eat the foods that were discouraged on previous diets and named unhealthy. It felt strange to me that I could eat something like a cheese omelette for my breakfast. The freedom to eat what felt like such an indulgence for breakfast, really suited me, especially as I've always been more of a savoury girl when it comes to food.

You might have heard the phrases 'clean' and 'dirty' when it comes to the keto diet. The clean keto diet, simply means that the focus of your diet is getting your nutrients from mainly fresh, unprocessed food. It follows the same makeup, in that it is low carb and high fat, but with the focus being on eating things that are as natural as they can be.

Some examples of foods you would eat on the clean keto diet are:

- Eggs
- Olive oil
- Fresh low carb fruits, such as strawberries
- Chicken
- Unprocessed meat
- Seafood

- Fresh vegetables- low carb of course, such as asparagus, cauliflower, broccoli and tomatoes

The bedrock of clean keto, is health. In eating this way, you'll enjoy the full range of benefits that come with being in ketosis, not to mention that you'll be fuelling your body with all of the nutrients that it needs.

However, eating this way costs money. The cost of living for most families is already high and rising. There is a certain amount of 'food snobbery' where clean eating is concerned. We should remember that eating 'clean' is a privilege that many families just don't have.

Dirty keto follows the same dietary principles; low carb and high fat but allows for processed foods and fast food as part of your diet. With dirty keto, you still eat the same macro ratios, but the focus isn't on food quality, but rather on convenience.

Dirty keto would include foods such as:

- Diet drinks
- Margarine
- Fast food
- Processed meats such as bacon and sausage
- Artificial sweeteners

- Processed cheese
- Low carb snack food such as pork scratchings

As with anything in life, it's about balance. I've never pretended to be one of those scary gym people, that eat quinoa and avocados, and run 10k every day. We are human beings with lives and good days and bad days. I try and live my life by the 80/20 ratio. If I can eat wholesome, nutrient rich, keto food for 80% of the time, then I certainly won't beat myself up for having a glass of wine and something from the 'dirty' list the other 20%. I urge you to do the same!

The combination of intermittent fasting and the keto diet is the entire focus of this book because it's the point when my life changed. Not only did I lose the weight I was trying to lose, but my hair loss slowed, my anxiety and depression lessened and I stopped having heart palpitations. I also regained my sex drive, much to my relief!

Another happy result of my keto diet with fasting was that I noticed a great deal of relief from my endometrial pain. I have suffered from endometriosis for many years and despite operations, I still suffer from symptoms. As the keto diet is so effective in helping with inflammatory conditions, I have noticed a massive reduction in my pain levels and an improvement in my mobility, after fasting with keto.

So, we know that intermittent fasting isn't just good for weight loss, but that it reduces inflammation **(Source 8)**, raises our levels of HGH **(Source 9)** and regulates our insulin levels. **(Source 10)**

Combining fasting and keto might seem like a lot of hard work, isn't fasting challenging enough on its own without adding a diet to it as well? Let's look at the benefits of doing both together:

- Enabling ketosis, faster- The wonderful thing about the keto diet, is how it naturally complements fasting. The aim of fasting is to use our body's glycogen stores up and to start burning fat. This is the focus of the keto diet! If you are already eating foods with a low carb diet, then your glycogen levels will already be low, thus leading to the fat burning stage sooner, helping your body to reach ketosis quicker. For those people that struggle to reach that point of ketosis while following the keto diet, adding the element of intermittent fasting can massively boost the process. This means that all of the benefits of fasting, the fat burning, the autophagy, the insulin regulation and the rise of HGH levels are all reached sooner. We should then enjoy the weight loss and with it, the reduction of our menopause symptoms.

- Stability- if we are eating low carb, then we don't have to switch between burning glycogen and fat all of the time.
- Appetite control- people that follow the keto diet experience a reduction in their appetite. This means that going for long periods of time without food will be easier. **(Source 11)**

Example Schedules of IF and Keto:

Here's what a typical day of combining keto and fasting might look like. As I follow the 16/8 method in my daily life, we'll use that as the example fasting window.

<u>Day 1</u>

7 am: Black coffee at intervals through the morning

1 pm: Fasting window closes

Lunch: 2 egg omelette made with cheese. A side of smoked salmon and a side salad of lettuce, tomato and cucumber

4 pm: Peppermint tea

7 pm: Dinner: Chicken stir-fry made with bok choi, ginger, garlic, broccoli, onion and red cabbage

8 pm: Evening snack: Ginger tea and a handful of walnuts and pecans

9 pm: Fasting window begins

Day 2

7 am: Black coffee at intervals throughout the morning

1 pm: Fasting window closes

Lunch: Tuna nicoise salad, with hard-boiled eggs, feta, lettuce and tomatoes

4 pm: Afternoon snack: A handful of olives

7 pm: Dinner: Roasted cauliflower steaks with a tomato and chilli salsa. Home-made Cajun spiced chicken thighs with lemon and garlic

8 pm: Evening snack: Camomile tea

9 pm: Fasting window opens

I mentioned before that my food tastes run to savoury, rather than sweet. However, if I do get a sweet craving,

I find that a handful of berries takes the craving away. As I don't have them very often, they taste super sweet to me, since doing keto and absolutely satisfy that craving.

Since following keto, I've found that I listen to my body's hunger signals better. On the days when I don't feel that hungry, I take the opportunity to do a 24 hr fast. This would mean that I would eat an evening meal on Day 1 as above, but then not eat again until the following evening on Day 2. I do this on average, twice a week. The key is to always listen to your body though. There are days when I wake up and can't wait until my eating window, I always say, if you cheat- make it keto! A shorter fasting window or a small snack won't ruin your hard work, a little flexibility might be the difference between sticking to plan or giving up!

Don't attempt keto and fasting together if you are one of the following:

- Under 18 years old
- Pregnant or trying to conceive
- Breastfeeding
- Suffer from type 1 diabetes- there is a risk of something called ketoacidosis where the PH of your body becomes too acidic because of

the high levels of ketones in your body. There are conflicting studies on this. My advice is to avoid)

- Have an eating disorder or a history of disordered eating- fasting and keto together are quite restrictive and it's easy to fall back into old habits and disorders.
- Are elderly
- Have a heart condition
- Have a kidney disorder

While most people should be able to happily fast and do keto together, as always there will be exceptions. Although the combination of the two provides a multitude of benefits, it is **crucial** to consult with your doctor or healthcare provider before you embark on a new diet.

When you start keto, there is a possibility of developing something commonly known as keto flu. This can manifest in the following ways:

- Headaches
- Nausea/upset stomach
- Dizziness
- Irritability
- Tiredness

Symptoms differ between people, some people don't get it at all, whereas others suffer badly and abandon the diet altogether.

Keto flu can happen for a couple of reasons. Most people have been eating a carb heavy diet, burning their glycogen stores as their primary energy source. When they stop eating carbs, their body is thrown off kilter while it switches to burning fat stores. Another reason is the drop in our insulin levels. When this happens we naturally lose salt and minerals out of our urine, causing dehydration and loss of important electrolytes. **(Source 12)** This can leave you feeling sluggish and foggy.

The good news is that most symptoms disappear after a few days, leaving you feeling better than ever. For a lot of people, it's hard to get over that hill though, especially when you feel rubbish.

Here are some top tips for getting through:

- Hydrate!- the keto diet causes you to lose your water stores because the glycogen stores bind themselves to water. **(Source 13)**When we lose the glycogen, the water goes with them! Keep drinking water to replenish your stores.

- Don't do high intensity exercise- your body is still adapting to a new source of energy, give yourself the time to gently adapt. However, low intensity exercise such as yoga or walking can be really beneficial.
- Replace your lost electrolytes- eating leafy greens and adding salt to your diet can help to replace those lost minerals.
- Get enough sleep- let yourself adapt gently and get plenty of rest
- Eat- make sure that you are eating enough!

The Mediterranean diet

The Mediterranean diet is another eating plan that works well alongside intermittent fasting. As I've said before, not all bodies are made the same and there are some people whose bodies react differently to low carb or high fat. The Mediterranean plan is a nice alternative to keto, which works well alongside fasting.

The Mediterranean diet isn't exactly a diet as such, but rather a way of eating that is inspired by the countries around the Mediterranean sea.

The focus of these country's diets are:
- Fresh fruit- Apples, bananas, oranges, peaches, figs, melon, pears, grapes and berries

- Vegetables- Tomatoes, broccoli, kale, spinach, cucumbers, potatoes, sweet potatoes, carrots
- Wholegrains- Wholegrain pasta, wild rice, wholegrain bread
- Nuts and seeds- Almonds, hazelnuts, cashews, chia seeds, pumpkin seeds and sunflower seeds
- Legumes- Beans, chickpeas, lentils and kidney beans
- Seafood- Fish and shellfish such as salmon, mussels, lobster, trout, mackerel and swordfish
- Eggs
- Poultry- Chicken, turkey and duck
- Olive oil and other healthy fats such as avocado oil

The diet also includes a small amount of alcohol, dairy and red meat, in moderation.

Although the focus is on fresh, you can still benefit from eating frozen and tinned vegetables.

What foods should you limit/avoid:
- Sugar- ice cream, fizzy drinks, cakes and chocolate. Try and get your sweet fix from

yoghurt and fruit. A small amount of dark chocolate is another option if you are having sweet cravings

- Processed meat- burgers, sausage, reformed meat, bacon, anything breaded or glazed. Some charcuterie meat such as parma ham is fine though
- Fast food- avoid anything deep fried in unhealthy oil, like fries
- Refined grains- white bread, white rice, white pasta, crisps
- Microwave meals- most of these are packed with sugars and additives
- Unhealthy fats- trans fats, saturated fats

There are many benefits of combining your fasting plan with the Mediterranean diet, which are:

- Personal taste- people's appetites and tastes vary a lot. A diet that is made up mainly of carbs and vegetables, without such a focus on meat, might appeal to people that want to be mindful of their meat consumption, or fit in better with vegetarianism or veganism.
- Potentially more sustainable- we know that the keto diet, for all its benefits, might be harder to follow and feel more restrictive.

The Mediterranean diet plan and fasting together can give you the benefits of fasting but without the super restrictive element that keto brings.

- Weight loss- Although the weight loss might not be as dramatic as it can be on keto, combining the Mediterranean diet with fasting can be good if steady weight loss is your goal. The diet plan itself is low in fat, with a focus on vegetables, protein and unprocessed foods. There is the risk that without specific guidelines on portion sizes and calories, you could lead to overeating. However, with the added element of a fasting window, this is unlikely. Even more reason to combine the two!

- Protects against Type 2 diabetes- following this eating style might help to stabilise blood sugar levels and protect you from the risk of type 2 diabetes. **(Source 14)**

- Cardiovascular benefits- research has shown that the Mediterranean diet is linked to lowering the risk of blood pressure, heart disease and strokes. **(Source 15)**

Here are some tips to help you combine the Mediterranean diet with intermittent fasting:

- Eat your protein- we know that eating protein keeps us fuller for longer, so combine your protein source with lots of fresh vegetables for extra impact.
- Use a tracking app- it might be helpful to use a food tracking app when doing a looser plan such as the Mediterranean diet not only to make sure you're getting a balanced selection of nutrients but to keep an eye on your calorie count.
- Eat seasonal- a great thing about the Mediterranean diet is the variety of food you can have. Make the most of it by fully exploring the variety of food choices available to you locally and seasonally.
- Get creative- choose new grains or vegetables to make exciting new meals with. You might still be limited on your eating window when you're fasting but your menu doesn't have to be. Make every meal count!

Chapter 7

Recipe Ideas

This chapter is going to give you inspiration with food for your keto/fasting journey. We've already talked about the difference between clean keto and dirty keto.

These recipes will be mainly based on the clean program, but I will throw a few recipes in that have 'dirty' elements or are completely dirty. These will be clearly marked so that there's no confusion though. We will also explore the Mediterranean diet and go through some recipes as an alternative to keto.

A lot of these recipes will specify almond flour. This is generally a quite expensive product, I've found that ground almonds are cheaper and usually more available in supermarkets. Almond flour has a finer texture, which some people tend to prefer. I've found that it works really well, but as with anything, it's down to personal taste.

It's also worth noting that not all sweeteners are keto friendly. There research to suggest that using sweeteners as a sugar replacement might discourage us from breaking the habits of high carb, high sugar that most of us fall into. However, I feel that it's better to use sweeteners to build ourselves eating plans that are sustainable. It's unrealistic to think that we will not want to eat sweet things. In my opinion, using sweeteners is a good way of sustaining these healthy new habits. As ever, you have to do what's best for you.

There are many sweeteners on the market, with varying degrees of suitability. As a rule, I'd recommend sticking to sweeteners derived from erythritol and stevia. These are both plant based and do not cause any sort of fluctuation in insulin. There are different varieties, with different textures, useful depending on what you're using them for.

Now let's get to the recipes for some inspiration.

Firstly, let's remind ourselves of the general foods that we can eat on keto.

Keto friendly foods:
- Meat- Beef, pork, lamb, goat, mutton
- Speciality meats- venison, rabbit
- Poultry- chicken, turkey, duck, goose
- Fish- Salmon, tuna, mackerel, cod, trout
- Seafood/Shellfish- prawns, crab, lobster- watch out for carb content in certain shellfish though, such as scallops
- Eggs

- Cheese- full fat cottage cheese, brie, camembert, manchego, gruyere, cheddar, goat's cheese Nothing processed though, or 'low fat'
- Nuts- almonds, walnuts, macadamia, brazil nuts etc.
- Seeds- chia, pumpkin, flaxseeds
- Healthy oils- olive oil, avocado oil,
- Avocados
- Vegetables- with a low carb content, tomatoes, peppers, onions, broccoli, cauliflower, turnip, bok choi
- Spices and herbs- oregano, onion powder, salt, pepper, thyme, ginger

Avoid 'diet' or 'low-fat' versions of things. On keto, fat is not to be feared! Often when low fat versions of foods are made, they add filler ingredients which can have higher amounts of carbs and sugar.

Let's talk about butter briefly. The carb content of butter is so low it's barely worth counting, to be exact it contains 0.009 grams. Many people that follow the 'clean' keto don't use butter because firstly, it's easy to overeat. Secondly, dairy is harder to digest and can lead to inflammation. Thirdly because there are plenty of butter alternatives, including ghee which is basically butter but with the lactose removed. There are also avocado oil, olive oil and coconut oils as alternatives. However, for the purposes of these recipes, I will be including heavy cream and butter as standard, they won't be labelled as 'dirty'.

What not to eat on Keto:

- All fruits- except for small portions of berries such as strawberries or blackberries
- Grains- rice, pasta, cereals
- Beans/legumes- kidney beans, chickpeas, lentils, peas
- Root veg- potatoes, carrots, parsnips, sweet potatoes
- Sugars- chocolate, cakes, biscuits
- Low fat/diet foods- mayonnaise, dressings, spreads, cheese
- Certain sauces- barbeque, ketchup, curry sauce, teriyaki
- Trans-fats- margarine, certain vegetable oils
- Alcohol- beer, wine, pre-mixed drinks
- Diet food- sweets, sweeteners, desserts

When I first began keto, I was totally overwhelmed by all of the new food rules, but give it time and you get the hang of it, I promise. Until you do, this chapter will go through every meal, giving you a mixture of keto recipe options.

Keto Breakfasts

Egg and Cheese Omelette: Serves 1

Prep time/ Cook time:
2 mins/5 mins

Ingredients:
2 eggs
10g cheddar cheese
½ tablespoon olive oil
salt and pepper
handful of chives

Method:
1. Break your eggs into a bowl, and season with salt and pepper
2. Roughly cut your chives and add to the egg mixture, mix well with a fork
3. Pop a small non-stick frying pan onto low heat to heat up
4. Grate your cheese and set aside
5. Add ½ tablespoon of olive oil to the pan
6. Gently pour your eggs into the pan and tilt the pan to spread the mixture around the pan
7. When the omelette begins to cook but is still raw in the middle, add the cheese to the middle of the mixture.

8. Use a non-stick spatula to gently lift the omelette, then fold it in half

9. It will be done when it turns golden brown

10. Plate up and enjoy!

Smoked Salmon and Scrambled Eggs: Serves 2

Prep time/ Cook time:

5 mins/5 mins

Ingredients:

200g smoked salmon

Salt and pepper

3 eggs

5 ml double cream

Dill sprigs

Method:

1. Break your eggs into a mixing bowl

2. Add seasoning and double cream and dill, reserving some dill for garnish

3. Put a non-stick pan on low heat

4. Cut your smoked salmon into strips

5. Add egg mixture to pan and stir gently

6. Add salmon and cook until eggs are set

7. Remove to a plate and top with dill sprigs to garnish

Soft Boiled Eggs with Avocado and Pancetta Soldiers: Serves 2

Prep time / Cook time:
5 mins / 5 -6 mins

Ingredients:
4 eggs (large)
1 avocado
100g pancetta

Method:
1. Bring a saucepan of water to a boil
2. Put the eggs into the water and boil for 5 minutes
3. Slice a de-stoned avocado and wrap each slice in pancetta
4. Fry for 2-3 minutes on high heat until crispy
5. Pop the eggs into egg cups and use the avocado pancetta soldiers to dip in your runny egg!

Breakfast Pockets: Serves 2-3

Prep time/ Cook time:
15 mins / 20-25 mins

Ingredients:
2 eggs (large)

2 ½ cups mozzarella (shredded)

1 cup of almond flour

2 oz cream cheese

½ teaspoon baking powder

Keto-friendly fillings- cheese, bacon etc

Method:

1. Preheat the oven to 180°C

2. Melt the mozzarella and the cream cheese together. Do this in 30-second blasts in the microwave so that it doesn't burn. Stir to combine

3. Add one of the eggs and stir in with the cheese

4. Whisk together the almond flour and baking powder in a separate bowl

5. Mix the two mixtures together and stir until a dough forms

6. Work the dough and divide it into balls. Pop onto baking paper and flatten the balls to make circles

7. Add your choice of fillings (not too full or they won't close)

8. Fold the dough over the filling and pinch the edges. Brush with the other egg (beaten)

9. Pop on a baking tray and bake for 20-25 mins until golden

Keto Pancakes: Serves 2

Prep time/ Cook time:

5 mins / 15 mins

Ingredients:

4 eggs

75 ml unsweetened almond milk

1 tsp sugar substitute

1 tsp baking powder

175g almond flour

½ tsp vanilla extract

pinch of cinnamon

Method:

1. Whisk the eggs and almond milk together in a bowl

2. Add sugar substitute, cinnamon, vanilla, baking powder, almond flour and combine

3. Pop a frying pan on medium heat and drop a small amount of batter into it

4. Cook for 2/3 mins until the edges are set. Turn them over and cook for another 3 mins until golden

3. Cook the remaining mixture and serve in stacks with your toppings

Keto English Muffins: Serves 1

Prep time/Cook time:

5 mins / 5 mins

Ingredients:

3 tbsp almond flour

½ tsp baking powder

1 tbsp melted butter

1 egg

Method:

1. Mix all ingredients together in a mug (a large mug is fine)
2. Cook in a microwave for 60-90 seconds
3. Cut in half and flatten them slightly so they're easier to toast
4. Toast in a toaster or fry in a pan

Egg Muffins: Makes 4

Prep time/Cook time:

5 mins / 15-20 mins

Ingredients:

3 eggs (large)

1-2 tbsp unsweetened almond milk

¼ tsp black pepper

½ cup of grated cheese

Fillings of your choice – I used bacon, onion and peppers and baby tomatoes

Method:

1. Pre heat oven to 190°C

2. In a jug, whisk the eggs and almond milk together.

3. Fry bacon, onions and peppers (Or fillings of your choice)

4. Grease or line a muffin tray. Put a sprinkle of each filling in the bottom of each muffin space

5. Pour over the egg mixture and sprinkle the top of each one with cheese

6. Bake at 190°C for 15-20 mins until golden

Stuffed Avocado Boats: Serves 1

Prep time/Cook time:

5 mins / 5 mins

Ingredients:

2 eggs (large)

1 avocado

20g cheddar

1 tsp black pepper

1 tsp sea salt

½ a red bell pepper, finely sliced

2 tsp chives (thinly sliced)

Method:

1. Preheat your oven to 200°C

2. Cut the avocados in half and remove the stone. Spoon a couple of tablespoons of avocado flesh out to make a well in it

3. Place the avocado halves cut side up onto an oven dish. Crack an egg into the centre

4. Sprinkle with salt and pepper

5. Bake for 6-7 mins. Sprinkle with cheese on top. Bake for a further 5-10 mins until they are cooked to your requirements

6. Sprinkle with chives and the diced peppers

Keto Cereal: Makes 6 portions

Prep time/Cook time:

5 mins/10 mins

Ingredients:

3 tbsp coconut oil

61g granulated sweetener

1 tsp cinnamon

1 tsp vanilla extract

½ tsp sea salt

130g coconut flakes

134g keto- friendly nuts such as hazelnuts, macadamia nuts

34g sunflower seeds

40g ground flaxseed

Method:

1. Line a baking sheet with baking paper

2. Melt the coconut oil in a pan over medium-high heat. Add sweetener and cinnamon and until all melted

3. Stir in the vanilla, salt, coconut, nuts, sunflower seeds, hemp seeds, and flaxseed

4. Stir evenly to coat with the coconut oil mixture

5. Reduce the heat to medium and toast the mixture. Cook for 4-5 mins until it's toasted not burnt

Serve with almond milk and blueberries

Keto Full English: Serves 1

Prep time/Cook time:

5 mins / 20-25 mins

Ingredients:

2 100% meat/gluten free sausages sausages

2-3 rashers of bacon

1 egg

2-3 mushrooms

1 tomato

Method:

1. Fry the sausages for 15-20 mins in a large frying pan

2. After 10 mins add bacon, mushrooms, and tomato halves

3. Lastly, when the rest of the ingredients are cooked, add the egg to the pan with a little oil if needed. Cook until the egg is ready and then serve!

Keto Lunches

Cucumber Boats: Serves 1

Prep time/Cook time:

5 mins / 4 mins

Ingredients:

1 cucumber

2 tablespoons full fat cream cheese

1 avocado

2 rashers of cooked bacon

chilli flakes

salt and pepper

Method:

132

1. Cook the bacon rashers until crispy and set aside
2. Cut the cucumber in half and scrape out the seeds, dry with a paper towel
3. Spread the cream cheese into the cucumber
4. Mash an avocado and add salt and pepper to it
5. Spread the avocado between the two cucumber halves
6. Crumble the bacon rashers and chilli flakes over the top and enjoy

Tomato Rings: Serves 1

Prep time/Cook time:
5 mins / 15 mins

Ingredients:
1 beef tomato
2 eggs
2 slices shredded ham
25g grated cheddar
handful of basil leaves
salt and pepper

Method:
1. Cut the tops off the tomato and discard
2. Cut the tomato into thick slices horizontally
3. Using a cutter or a knife, cut out the middle of the tomato leaving a thick ring of tomato that looks like an onion ring

4. Set aside the tomato middles and shred the ham and basil

5. Crack the eggs and mix

6. Heat a pan with butter until fairly hot

7. Take the tomato middles, egg, and ham and mix together with the basil leaves, season with salt and pepper

8. Lay the tomato rings in the buttery pan and cook for a few minutes

9. Pour the egg mixture into the tomato rings so the mixture is contained within and gently fry. Add the cheese on top

10. After 5-7 mins, turn over and repeat the process

11. Serve with basil leaves to garnish

Halloumi and Bacon Salad: Serves 1

Prep time/Cook time:
5 mins / 10 mins

Ingredients:
2 slices halloumi
2 rashers bacon
¼ iceberg lettuce
Spinach leaves (about a handful)
3-4 cherry tomatoes
2 leaves of raw cabbage
1 tbsp olive oil

1-2 tsp of chopped onion

6 green olives

1-2 slices of cheddar cheese

2 tsp of full fat mayonnaise

Method:

1. Heat oil in a pan over medium heat

2. Add the bacon and halloumi and cook for 3-5 mins, turning halfway. Cook until golden

3. Set aside to cool

4. Chop all ingredients to your desired size and add t0 a large bowl

5. Add your bacon and halloumi and serve with mayonnaise

<u>Slow Cooker Meaty Cabbage soup:</u>
<u>Serves 6</u>

Prep time/Cook time:

30 mins / 5-8 hours

Ingredients:

450g pork mince

450g beef mince

1 small onion, chopped

4-5 garlic cloves, finely chopped

1 regular size tin of chopped tomatoes

2 tsp dried oregano

2 tsp dried thyme

1 tsp cumin

1 tsp chilli flakes

1 small green cabbage, chopped

1 litre liquid beef stock

salt and pepper

Method:

1. Heat the oil in a pan over medium heat and saute onion and garlic until the onion becomes translucent

2. Add the pork and beef mince

3. Cook until the meat is no longer pink

4. Add the meat and onion mixture into the slow cooker.

5. Add all of the herbs, spices, salt and pepper and tomatoes into the slow cooker. Add the beef stock and cabbage

6. Cook for 4-5 hours on high, or 7-8 hours on low

This can be adapted if you don't have a slow cooker. Use a hob to follow steps 1-5. Bring the mixture to a boil, then reduce the heat and simmer for 25-30 mins until the cabbage is soft.

Bacon and Mushroom Quiche: 8 servings

Prep time/Cook time:

10 mins/1 hour

Ingredients:

The crust:
262g of almond flour
½ tsp sea salt
56g of butter
1 large egg

The filling:
5 large eggs
79ml of almond milk or double cream
25g cooked onion
165g cooked mushrooms
115g cooked bacon
235g cheddar cheese
½ tsp salt
¼ tsp pepper

Method:
1. Preheat oven to 180°C. Line a 9-inch quiche dish with baking paper or grease it
2. In a bowl, mix all the crust ingredients until it's all combined and looks like a dough
3. Using two pieces of baking paper, spray the bottom one with oil, place dough between them and roll out the dough until ¼ inch thick
4. Place over the prepared dish and slide the parchment away. It may slightly fall apart, just push the dough back

into place. Prick crust with a fork to prevent bubbling and cook for approx 10 mins until lightly golden. Allow to cool for 15 mins before adding the filling

5. Place the cooked onion, mushrooms and bacon over the bottom of the base making sure there is an even amount of each all over

6. Mix the eggs, milk substitute and salt and pepper together, then stir in the cheese

7. Pour over the bacon mixture, making sure the cheese is evenly distributed

8. Place tin foil over the quiche crust to prevent it from burning

9. Bake for approximately 30-35 mins until set

Keto Pizza: Serves 1

Prep time/Cook time:
10 mins / 25 mins

Ingredients:
1 egg
2 tbsp full fat cream cheese
24 g almond flour
336g of shredded mozzarella
½ tsp garlic powder
½ tsp mixed herbs
Keto- friendly toppings of your choice.

Method:

1. Put mozzarella and cream cheese into a microwavable bowl and heat for 90 seconds, stirring after 60 seconds

2. Stir again to make sure it's all combined and then add the egg and almond flour.

3. Mix well

4. Spread the mixture thinly onto an oven sheet lined with baking paper
(use wet hands to prevent sticking)

5. Poke holes with a fork to stop it from bubbling

6. Sprinkle with the herbs and garlic powder

7. Cook in the oven at 200°C for 10-15 mins
checking for bubbles. If bubbles appear then poke them with a fork

8. Top with the toppings of your choice and bake again until golden and crispy

Loaded Lettuce Lunch Wraps: Serves 2

Prep time/Cook time:
5 mins / 5mins

Ingredients:
4 lettuce leaves, whole
4 rashers of bacon
1 avocado
1 large tomato

mayonnaise

chives

Method:

1. Wash 4 lettuce leaves and dry them with kitchen towel

2. Fry bacon until crispy and set aside

3. De-stone and slice the avocado. Slice the tomato and dice the chives

4. Spread mayonnaise onto the lettuce and assemble the ingredients on top

5. Roll the lettuce into wraps

Broccoli and Stilton Soup: Serves 4

Prep time/Cook time:

10 mins / 25-30 mins

Ingredients:

Large head of broccoli, cut into florets

220g stilton

1 stick of celery

1 leek

20g butter

1 litre of gluten free vegetable stock

1 small head of cauliflower, cut into florets

2 tbsp olive oil

Method:

1. Heat a pan and add olive oil. Gently sauté the onion until translucent

2. Slice the celery and leek and add to the pan with the butter. Let this sweat for 5 mins

3. Pour in the stock and cook for 10-15 mins until everything is soft

4. Add the cauliflower and broccoli and cook for another 10 mins

5. Blitz in a blender or use a hand blender until it reaches your desired consistency

6. Stir in the stilton and allow the heat of the soup to melt it

7. Season if needed

Mushroom Soup: Serves 4

Prep time/ Cook time:

5 mins/25 mins

Ingredients:

500g mushrooms, sliced

100g leek, sliced

100g onion, sliced

salt and pepper

20g of butter

1 litre of chicken stock

Method

1. Heat butter in a saucepan and saute the onion and leek over gentle heat

2. Add the mushrooms

3. Add the chicken stock, the salt and pepper and simmer for 20 mins

4. Blend in a blender or use a hand blender until it gets to your desired consistency

Chaffles: Serves 1

Prep time/ Cook time:
5 mins/5-10 mins

Ingredients:
1 egg (large)
½ tsp salt
169 g mozzarella

You'll need a mini waffle iron for this one!

Method:

1. Whisk the egg, salt and add half of the cheese

2. Heat up the mini waffle iron and sprinkle a little bit of cheese on the bottom of the iron

3. Pour half of the mixture onto the iron and add a little bit more cheese

4. Cook for 2-3 mins until golden

5. Cook the other half of the mixture

6. Leave to cool and crisp up

Keto Dinners

Keto Chicken Fajitas: Serves 2

Prep time/ Cook time:

10 mins/ 25 mins

Ingredients:

Iceberg lettuce leaves

1 tsp chilli powder

1 tsp paprika

1 tsp oregano

1 tsp ground cumin

½ tsp salt

3 chicken breasts

1 red pepper

1 onion

2 garlic cloves

60 ml olive oil

1 tbsp lime juice

sour cream to garnish

handful of coriander

Method:

1. Slice the chicken breasts, the pepper and the onion into long strips
2. Finely dice the garlic
3. Mix the chilli powder, paprika, oregano, cumin, and salt in a small bowl and set aside
4. Put the chicken and the vegetables into a bowl and add the oil, the lime juice and the spices on top. Mix well
5. Line a baking tray and set the oven to 200°C
6. Spread the mixture out onto the tray and bake for 20-25 mins
7. Take the larger leaves from the iceberg and use them in place of a wrap to make fajitas. Garnish with coriander and sour cream

Butter Chicken: Serves 4

Prep time/ Cook time:

4 hours/30 mins

Ingredients:

800g chicken breast

4 garlic cloves (2 finely crushed, 2 finely chopped)

2cm ginger, peeled and finely grated

½ tsp fine sea salt

½ tsp hot chilli powder

1½ tbsp lemon juice

75ml natural yoghurt

½ tsp garam masala

½ tsp ground turmeric

1 tsp ground cumin

1-2 tbsp olive oil

1½ tbsp melted butter

2cm ginger, peeled and finely chopped

1 cardamom pod, seeds lightly crushed

2 cloves

1 tsp ground coriander

1 tsp garam masala

1 tsp ground turmeric

1 tsp hot chilli powder

275ml tomato puree

1 tbsp lemon juice

40g unsalted butter

100ml double cream

1 tbsp chopped coriander

This recipe is based on Gordon Ramsey's butter chicken, but with a few tweaks to make it keto friendly. It's one of the best, most flavourful Indian dishes I've ever made. Don't rush the prep side, it's worth taking a bit more time with it.

Method:

1. Place the chicken in a bowl with the garlic, ginger, salt, chilli powder and lemon juice. Mix, cover with cling film and chill for 30 mins

2. Mix together the yogurt, garam masala, turmeric and cumin and add to the chicken, making sure that each piece is well coated with the mixture. Cover again and chill for 3-4 hours

3. Heat your oven to 180 °C. Put the marinated chicken pieces on a grill rack set on a baking tray and bake for 8-10 mins. Brush the chicken pieces with a little olive oil and turn them over

4. Bake for another 10-12 mins until just cooked through

For the sauce:

1. Heat 1 ½ tsp of the butter in a pan and add the garlic and ginger

2. Fry for a min or so then add the cardamom, cloves, coriander, garam masala, turmeric and chilli powder

3. Stir well and fry for 1-2 mins. Stir in the tomato puree and lemon juice and cook for another couple of mins

4. Add the chicken pieces to the sauce and stir well to coat

5. Finally, add the butter and cream and stir continuously until the butter has melted and the sauce is smooth

6. Transfer to a warm bowl and serve hot, garnished with chopped coriander

Courgette Lasagne: Serves 6

Prep time/ Cook time:
10 mins / 45 mins

Ingredients:
400g courgette
2 tbsp olive oil
1 onion finely chopped
2 garlic cloves, finely chopped
650g minced beef
1 tbsp dried basil
1 tbsp dried oregano
1 tsp salt
¼ tsp ground black pepper
4 tbsp tomato puree
3 tbsp water

For the sauce:
350 ml heavy whipping cream
230 g shredded cheese, divided
1 garlic clove, minced
salt and black pepper to taste

Method:

1. Preheat the oven to 200°C

2. Thinly slice the courgettes lengthwise

3. Lay the courgette slices on paper towels and lightly sprinkle them with salt. Rest for 10 minutes and then pat dry with paper towels

4. Heat the olive oil in a large frying pan, over medium heat. Add the onion and garlic, and sauté until soft

5. Add the beef, basil, oregano, salt, and pepper. Stir together and cook until lightly browned

6. Stir in the tomato puree and water until well combined

7. Reduce the temperature to medium-low, and simmer for 5-10 minutes stirring occasionally

8. Add the cream, half of the cheese and the garlic to a medium-sized saucepan. Bring to a simmer over medium-high heat, and once bubbling, reduce the temperature to medium-low

9. Simmer for about 5 minutes while stirring continuously until the sauce has thickened. Season to taste

10. Assemble the lasagne by spreading about 1/3 of the meat sauce on the bottom of the baking dish that measures 10×8 inches

11. Cover with some of the cheese sauce and then cover with courgette slices on top, in a single layer. Repeat the layers and finish by sprinkling the remaining cheese on top

12. Bake in the oven for about 18-20 minutes or until the cheese is golden and bubbly

Chicken and Vegetable Curry Soup: Serves 4

Prep time/ Cook time:

10 mins/ 4 hr 30 mins

Ingredients:

2 tbsp olive oil

4 chicken thighs, skin removed

1 onion, chopped

3-4 garlic cloves, finely chopped

1 heaped tsp pureed ginger

8-10 closed cup mushrooms, chopped

1 large carrot sliced

1 celery stick, cut in half lengthways and chopped

6 brussel sprouts, ends removed, outer leaves removed and then chopped

¼ small white cabbage chopped

1-2 tbsp mild/medium/hot curry powder (depending on taste!)

1 heaped tsp paprika

1-2 tsp mild chilli powder

½ tsp black paper

1 tbsp dried coriander

250g passata

800ml chicken stock (I used 2 stock cubes)

400g can coconut milk

Small broccoli head cut into small florets

1 green pepper/capsicum, deseeded and cut into 1-2 inches pieces

Method:

1. Preheat oven to 160°C

2. In an oven proof casserole pot, over medium heat, add oil and cook the onion for 3-5 minutes until soft

3. Add the garlic and ginger and cook for a further 2-3 minutes. Add mushrooms and cook for 3-4 minutes, then add carrots, brussel sprouts and cabbage and cook for another 2-3 minutes, stirring

4. Add the chicken and cook for 1-2 mins on each side making sure they are on the bottom of the pot

5. Add the herbs and spices and stir

6. Add passata, then enough chicken stock to cover chicken and vegetables

7. Bring up to a boil and then put in the oven with the lid on for 4 hours

8. Put back on the hob over a medium heat and add the coconut milk, broccoli and peppers and mix well

9. Simmer for 10 minutes or until the broccoli is cooked to your liking

10. Serve with cauliflower rice or in a bowl on its own

Chicken and Prawn Keto style pad Thai:
Serves 1-2

Prep time/ Cook time:

5 mins/20 mins

Ingredients:

2 garlic cloves, finely chopped

½ 1 tsp chilli flakes depending on your taste

large handful of bean sprouts

large handful of stir-fry vegetables (thinly sliced carrot, cabbage, onion etc)

1 chicken breast, thinly sliced

2 eggs beaten

sesame oil

low carb noodles (I used bare naked noodles, which are 1g of carbs per serving)

40g cooked prawns

handful of chopped keto friendly nuts

1 tbsp soy sauce

Method:

1. Cook chicken in the oil for 5 mins until cooked through

2. Add garlic and cook for 1-2 mins.

3. Add bean sprouts and vegetables and cook for 4-5 mins

4. Push to one side or put in a separate frying pan.

5. Heat more oil and cook eggs while stirring until it looks like scrambled eggs

6. Mix with other ingredients and add drained noodles. Cook for 1-2 mins

7. Add prawns, nuts and soy sauce and cook for another 2-3 mins until prawns are heated through. (Be careful not to overcook them)

Fish Curry: Serves 2

Prep time/ Cook time:
5 mins/25 mins

Ingredients:
1 tbsp oil
1 onion, chopped
1 garlic clove, crushed
1 tbsp curry powder
1 tsp turmeric
1 tsp garam masala
1 and ½ tsp chilli flakes
400ml can coconut milk
390g white fish (Cut into chunks. You can use any firm white fish, salmon fillet or raw prawns)

Method:

1. Heat the oil in a large deep frying pan or saucepan over medium heat

2. Add the onion and a small pinch of salt

3. Gently fry for approximately 5-8 minutes until the onion is translucent, then add the garlic and spices.

4. Stir and cook for another minute, adding a splash of water to prevent them from sticking. Tip in the coconut milk and stir well, then simmer for 10 mins.

5. Tip the fish into the pan and cook for approximately 3-4 minutes until the fish is starting to flake. Season to taste. Ladle into bowls and serve with cauliflower rice. (See side dishes)

(You can also do this with chicken. Just cook the chicken first before adding the other ingredients)

Peanut Butter Chicken: Serves 8

Prep time/ Cook time:
10 mins / 45 mins

Ingredients:
2 tbsp coconut oil
8 skinless boneless chicken thighs
1 onion, chopped
3 garlic cloves, crushed
2 red chillies (finely slices and deseeded)

2 tsp fresh ginger- grated

2 tbsp garam masala

100g smooth peanut butter (check sugar levels!)

400 ml coconut milk

400g chopped tomatoes

1 tbsp coriander

roasted peanuts to serve

cauliflower rice to serve

Method:

1. Heat 1 tbsp of the oil in a deep frying pan over a medium heat

2. Brown the chicken in batches, setting aside once cooked and golden

3. Fry the onion for 5-8 minutes until softened. Add the garlic, chilli and ginger and fry in the remaining oil for 1 min

4. Add the garam masala and fry for 1 min more

5. Stir in the peanut butter, coconut milk and tomatoes, and bring to a simmer

6. Return the chicken to the pan and add the chopped coriander. Cook for 30 mins until the sauce thickens

7. Serve with the remaining coriander, roasted peanuts and cauliflower rice

Lemon and Garlic Chicken: Serves 2-3

Prep time/ Cook time:

2hr 10 mins/15 mins

Ingredients:

1 lemon, juiced

2 tbsp olive oil

1 teaspoon Dijon mustard

2 garlic cloves minced

¼ tsp salt

1/8 tsp black pepper

4 skin-on, bone-in chicken thighs

4 lemon wedges

Method:

1. Whisk the oil, lemon, mustard, salt and pepper and garlic and pop in a bowl

2. Place the chicken into a bowl or a plastic bag. Pour marinade over the chicken and seal the bowl or the bag

3. Refrigerate for at least 2 hours

4. Remove the chicken from the marinade and pat dry with paper towels.

5. Fry in a pan on medium heat turning, for 15 mins until the juices run clear

You can also do this in an airfryer or on a baking sheet in the oven. Serve with the cauliflower rice and the tomato and coriander salsa.

Sea Bass with Ginger and Garlic: Serves 3

Prep time/ Cook time:

15 mins / 10 mins

Ingredients:

3 sea bass fillets

3 tbsp olive oil

small piece of ginger, peeled and sliced

1 ½ garlic cloves, thinly sliced

1 ½ red chillies, seeds removed and sliced thinly

2 or 3 spring onions, cut lengthways

1 tbsp soy sauce

Method:

1. Make 3 cuts in the skin of the fillets and season with salt and pepper

2. Add olive oil to a frying pan and when hot, place the fillets in and fry for 5 mins, with the skin side down

3. Turn the fillets over and cook for another minute

4. Remove fillets to a warm plate

5. Heat 2 tbsp olive oil, fry the chilli, ginger and garlic until softened

6. Add the spring onions and cook for a further minute with the soy sauce

7. Spoon mixture over the fish and serve

Spaghetti Bolognese with Zoodles: Serves 3-4

Prep time/ Cook time:
5 mins/30-45 mins

Ingredients:
500g mince beef
2 onions
2 tbsp olive oil
500g mushrooms
2 garlic cloves
500ml low carb beef stock
2 tins of chopped tomatoes
1 tsp oregano
1 tsp dried basil
4 tsp tomato puree
Basil leaves
Sprinkling of cheddar cheese
5 courgettes- or you can buy ready-made zoodles, the choice is yours!

Method:

1. Heat the olive oil and fry the minced beef until brown

2. Chop the onions, garlic and mushrooms and add them to the mince

3. When the veg is soft, add the tinned tomatoes, the beef stock and spices

4. Leave to simmer for 30-40 mins until the liquid reduces

5. In the meantime, if you are making your own zoodles, take the courgettes and use a spiralizer to create the zoodles.

6. Line a baking tray with a baking sheet and spread the zoodles out. Bake for about 15 mins at 180°C

7. Serve with the bolognese and sprinkle with some cheddar cheese

Side Dishes

Keto Coleslaw: 8 servings

Prep time/Cook time:
5 mins/10 mins

Ingredients:
350g green cabbage, thinly sliced
170g red cabbage, thinly sliced
2 spring onions, thinly sliced
5g cup parsley

77g full fat mayonnaise

2 tbsp sour cream

2 tsp apple cider vinegar

2 tsp lemon juice

¼ tsp garlic powder

¼ tsp salt

pinch of pepper

Method:

1. Mix together the cabbages, spring onions and parsley and toss in a large bowl

2. Add the remaining ingredients into a second bowl and mix together until smooth

3. Pour half the dressing into the cabbage bowl and mix well

Keto Onion Rings: Makes 4 Servings

Prep time/ Cook time:

5 mins / 15-20 mins

Ingredients:

1 large onion

1 egg

1 pinch of salt

1 tbsp olive oil

½ tbsp paprika

1 tsp garlic powder

50g almond flour

45g parmesan

Method:

1. Preheat an oven to 200°C

2. Slice the onion into rings

3. Mix the dry ingredients into a bowl

4. Beat the egg in another bowl

5. Dip the onion rings into the egg and then into the dry ingredients bowl

6. Drizzle the olive oil over the onion rings and bake on a baking sheet for 15-20 mins until golden

Garlic and Parmesan Roasted Asparagus: Makes 4 Servings

Prep time/ Cook time:

5 mins/8 mins

Ingredients:

226g fresh asparagus

½ tsp salt

½ tsp fresh ground black pepper

3 garlic cloves, minced

2-3 tbsp parmesan cheese

olive oil spray

Method:

1. Preheat oven to 220°C

2. Line a baking tray with baking paper and set aside

3. Rinse the asparagus and trim off woody end pieces

4. Spread them out evenly on a baking sheet

5. Spray the asparagus lightly with a coat of olive oil spray

6. Sprinkle with salt, pepper, garlic, and parmesan cheese. Use your hands to mix the asparagus with all of the ingredients, then lay it out into an even layer again. Spray with one more light coat of olive oil

7. Bake in the preheated oven for 8 minutes

8. Remove from oven and serve immediately

Cauliflower Rice: Serves 2-4

Prep time/ Cook time:
5 mins / 5 mins

Ingredients:
Cauliflower
Sesame oil

You can buy frozen cauliflower rice but I have found it to be quite wet and soft so I prefer to make my own as it's really easy. I also tend to use a whole cauliflower and put what I don't need in an airtight container. It can last 3-5 days in the fridge.

Method:
1. Put the florets into a food blender and blitz for approximately 30 seconds until it evenly resembles rice. (I often give it a bit of a stir after 10-15 seconds)
2. Heat some oil (I like sesame seed oil for a nutty taste if having it with a curry) and add the cauliflower rice
3. Cook for 3-5 minutes and serve

Marmite Brussels Sprouts: Serves 8

Prep time/Cook time:
10 mins / 10 mins

Ingredients:
100g unsalted butter
500g sprouts
3 tsp marmite

Method:
1. Beat the butter and the marmite together. Decant into a pot, or roll into a log and chill
2. Halve the sprouts and boil them for 3-4 minutes
3. Drain the sprouts and leave them to steam dry

4. Heat a frying pan, add the sprouts and dry fry them for 4-5 mins until they start to blacken on the edges and sides

5. Remove from the heat and add a chunk of the marmite butter

6. Shake the pan to coat them and season with pepper

Cauliflower Roasties: Serves 3

Prep time/Cook time:
5 mins/20mins

Ingredients:
1 cauliflower
cut into small florets (the smaller they are, the quicker they will cook)
100g butter, sliced thinly

So quick and simple! The texture of roast potatoes but minus the carbs! Roasting it in butter infuses cauliflower with a nutty flavour that is simply delicious!

Method:
1. Preheat the oven to 200c
2. Put the cauliflower in a baking dish, season with salt and pepper to taste and cover with slices of butter
3. Bake for approximately 20 minutes, depending on the size of the florets

Mexican Rice: Serves 2-3

Prep time/ Cook time:

10 mins/20 mins

Ingredients:

½ a cauliflower

1 tbsp olive oil

½ onion, chopped

½ jalapeno pepper

2 garlic cloves, crushed

2 tbsp tomato puree

1 tsp cumin

1 tsp salt

2 tbsp finely diced coriander

Method:

1. Blitz the cauliflower in a food processor into the rice. (You can use frozen but fresh has a better texture)

2. Heat the oil in a frying pan on medium heat

3. When the oil is hot add the onion and jalapeno and cook for approx 5 mins until softened

4. Add the garlic and tomato puree and cook for a further 1 min

5. Add the cauliflower rice, cumin and salt and cook over medium heat, stirring occasionally, for 5 minutes or until the cauliflower is as soft as you'd like

6. Stir in the coriander just before serving

Cauliflower Potato Salad: Serves 4

Prep time/ Cook time:
5 mins/15 mins

Ingredients:
1 tbsp olive oil
1 lb cauliflower, cut into florets
77g mayonnaise
2 tbsp white vinegar
1 tsp garlic powder
¼ tsp paprika
¼ tsp celery salt
¼ tsp sea salt
¼ tsp pepper
1 tbsp dijon mustard
2 hard-boiled eggs, chopped
13 g chopped red onion
26g spring onions, chopped

Method:
1. Cook the cauliflower until fork tender, for about 10 minutes
2. Cool to room temperature for 20-30 minutes

3. Whisk the rest of the ingredients together except for the onion, eggs and spring onions

4. Stir the dressing in the bowl with the cauliflower then add the remaining ingredients

5. Chill for 30 minutes or until ready to serve

<u>Turnip Fries: 8 Servings</u>

Prep time/Cook time:
15 mins / 30 mins

Ingredients:
8 turnips
3 tbsp olive oil
20g grated Parmesan cheese
1 ½ tsp garlic salt
1 tsp paprika
1 tsp onion powder

Method:
1. Peel and chop the turnips into fry shapes

2. Pop the turnip fries into a bowl and pour the oil into the bowl. Toss the fries to coat them well

3. Add the spices and the parmesan into a separate bowl

4. Sprinkle the spice mix over the fries and toss again so they are well coated

6. Bake at 200°C on a lined baking sheet for 20 mins

7. Turn them over and then cook for another 10 mins until crispy

Roasted Artichokes: Serves 4

Prep time/ Cook time:
15 mins/30 mins

Ingredients:
3 artichokes
2 tbsp olive oil
½ tsp salt
½ tsp black pepper
5 garlic cloves
1 lemon, sliced into rounds
1 tbsp butter

Method:
1. Trim the top and bottoms of the artichokes
2. Remove the sharp outer leaves
3. Cut the artichokes lengthways in half
4. Rub them with a slice of lemon to prevent burning
5. Use a spoon to remove the middle section of the artichokes
6. Place the artichokes cut-side up onto a baking tray, sprinkle with salt and pepper and then brush with olive oil

7. Fill the middle section with garlic cloves and lemon rounds then season with salt and pepper

8. Bake for 15 mins then turn over and brush again with olive oil. Cook for a further 10-15 mins

Roasted Keto Vegetables: Serves 3-4

Prep time/ Cook time:

10 mins/ 20-25 mins

Ingredients:

1 medium head of broccoli

1 medium cauliflower

2 courgettes

1 red onion

4 garlic cloves

1 green pepper

1 red pepper

4 tbsp of olive oil

2 tbsp balsamic vinegar

1 tsp garlic pepper

1 tsp oregano

1 tsp dried basil

1 tsp sea salt

1 tsp pepper

Method:

1. Preheat oven to 220°C

2. Cut the broccoli and cauliflower into smaller pieces

3. Cut the onions, courgettes and peppers into 2-3 cm chunks and decant onto a lined baking tray

4. Mix the olive oil with the balsamic and the herbs and spices and pour over the vegetables, mixing well

5. Leave the garlic cloves unpeeled and put them in with the vegetables

6. Bake for 20-25 mins until vegetables are roasted and golden

Desserts

<u>Blueberry Swirl Cheesecake: 8 Servings</u>

Prep time/ Cook time:

20 mins / 45 mins

Ingredients:

Almond crumb base:

100g ground almonds/almond flour

1 tbsp sugar alternative (I used truvia in this case)

57g butter

Filling:

340g full fat cream cheese

35g sugar alternative

2 tbsp fresh lemon juice

1 tsp lemon zest

pinch salt

240 ml heavy whipping cream

For the swirl:

190g frozen blueberries

1 tbsp sugar alternative

1 ½ -2 tbsp water

1/4 tsp xanthan gum

Method:

1. In a mixing bowl, place all the dry base ingredients and stir to combine. Add the melted butter to form a crumb mix

2. With greaseproof paper, line an 8×8" baking pan

3. Into the bottom, press the base mix to get neat edges, smooth with the back of a spoon

For the filling:

1. Add the zest, sugar alternative, lemon juice, cream cheese and salt into a bowl

2. Mix with an electric mixer for approx 1 min until combined. Adjust the sweetness to your liking.

3. Whip the cream in a separate bowl until it gets thick (don't over whisk it or it gets stiff and won't fold in)

4. With a spatula, fold the cream through the cream cheese to combine

For the swirl:

1. Add the frozen berries, sugar alternative and water in a small saucepan

2. Simmer this on medium heat for about 5 minutes, until the sauce thickens. With the back of a spoon/spatula, you can squash some of the blueberries

3. Turn off the heat, add the xanthan gum and allow it to fully cool

To assemble:

1. On top of the base, spoon the cheesecake filling and with a silicone spatula, smooth the top

2. Add dollops of cooled blueberries and with a toothpick/tip of a sharp knife, swirl to make a pattern

3. To fully set, place in a fridge, for about 8 hours/overnight

4. Place into the freezer, about an hour before serving to firm up and to make slicing easier. With a sharp knife, slice into 8 bar shapes

Cookies and Cream: Makes 12

Prep time/ Cook time:
15 mins/20 mins

Ingredients:
For cookie crumbles:
120g almond flour

3 tbsp cocoa powder

½ tsp salt

3 tbsp granulated sugar alternative

4 tbsp melted butter

2 tsp pure vanilla extract

For the filling:

28g cream cheese, softened

120 ml heavy cream

3 tbsp granulated sugar alternative

1 can coconut cream

1 tsp pure vanilla extract

Method:

1. Line a muffin tin with cupcake liners and spray with non-stick cooking spray

2. In a non-stick frying pan over medium heat, toast almond flour, mixing constantly until golden

3. Whisk in cocoa powder, salt, and sugar alternative. Mix in the melted butter and vanilla extract

4. Fill each liner with a heaped tablespoon of the chocolate cookie mixture, pressing it with the back of a spoon

5. Place the remaining mixture into the freezer for 20 minutes.

6. Using a hand mixer or whisk, mix the cream cheese, heavy cream, sugar alternative, coconut cream and vanilla until fluffy and thick

7. Divide the mixture evenly on top of the cookie mixture and crumble the frozen cookie mixture over top. Freeze for at least 3 hours before serving

Ice-cream: Makes 8 Servings

Prep time/ Cook time:
5 mins / 8 ½ hours

Ingredients:
2 cans coconut milk (15 oz)
480 ml of heavy cream
25g of sugar alternative
1 tsp pure vanilla extract
A pinch of salt

Method:
1. Chill coconut milk in the fridge for at least 3 hours, ideally overnight
2. Make whipped coconut: Spoon coconut cream into a large bowl, leaving the liquid in can, and use a hand mixer to beat coconut cream until very creamy. Set aside
3. In a separate large bowl using a hand mixer (or in a bowl of a stand mixer), beat heavy cream until soft peaks form. Beat in sweetener and vanilla
4. Fold whipped coconut into whipped cream, then transfer mixture into a loaf pan tin

5. Freeze until solid for about 5 hours

Chocolate Mug Cake: Serves 1

Prep time/ Cook time:

5 mins / 1 min

Ingredients:

2 tbsp butter

25g almond flour

2 tbsp cocoa powder

1 large egg, beaten

2 tbsp keto friendly chocolate chips

2 tbsp granulated sugar alternative

½ tsp baking powder

Pinch of salt

2 tbsp of whipped cream, for serving (optional)

Method:

1. Place butter in a microwave-safe mug and heat until melted this should take about 30 seconds

2. Add remaining ingredients except whipped cream and stir until fully combined

3. Cook for 45 seconds to 1 minute, or until cake is set but still fudgey

4. Top with whipped cream to serve

Chocolate Mousse: Serves 2

Prep time/ Cook time:
15 mins/5 mins plus time to chill

Ingredients:
355ml cups double cream
30g unsweetened cocoa powder
25g sugar alternative
½ tsp unsweetened vanilla extract

Method:
1. Chill the cream and put into a large mixing bowl
2. Use a mixer to whip the cream until stiff peaks form
3. Add remaining ingredients and whip until it forms a smooth mousse texture
4. Divide into 2 small bowls and serve

Coconut Balls: 10 Servings

Prep time/ Cook time:
10 mins/35 mins

Ingredients:
6 tbsp butter
42g finely shredded coconut
1 tsp cardamom
½ tsp vanilla extract

1 tsp ground cinnamon

Method:
1. Mix together the butter, half of the shredded coconut and spices in a bowl
2. Put the mixture into a bowl and refrigerate for 5-10 mins until firm
3. When they are chilled, roll into balls and roll in the remaining coconut

Fruit Platter And Nut Platter: Serves 1

Prep time/ Cook time:
5 mins /-

Ingredients:
Strawberries
Blackberries
Blueberries
Raspberries
Macadamia nuts
Hazelnuts
Almonds
Walnuts

Method:
1. Assemble your fruit any way you like and serve with nuts and a spoonful of the keto ice-cream

Strawberries and Cream: Serves 1

Prep time/ Cook time:
5 mins /-

Ingredients:
½ punnet of strawberries
125 ml of pouring cream
sprinkling of sugar substitute

Method:
1. Hull your strawberries and pop into a bowl
2. Pour on your cream and sprinkle a little sugar substitute on and enjoy

Peanut Butter Fudge: Makes 24 Pieces

Prep time/ Cook time:
5 mins/7 hours

Ingredients:
240g sugar-free peanut butter
113g unsalted butter
2 tsp vanilla extract

200g powdered sugar-substitute

¼ tsp salt

Method:

1. Line an 8-inch square baking tin with baking paper, make sure it goes up and over the sides

2. Combine the peanut butter and butter in a mixing bowl

3. Cover the bowl and microwave for a minute at a time, until the butter is melted

4. Remove the bowl from the microwave and add the vanilla and salt and stir until the mixture is combined

5. Add in the sugar alternative and stir until well mixed

6. Transfer the fudge into the tin and smooth the top with a spatula

7. Chill overnight or for at least 7 hours

8. When suitably chilled, remove from pan and cut up into 24 squares

Keto Lemon Bars: Makes 8

Prep time/ Cook time:

10 mins/ 1 hr

Ingredients:

114g melted butter

172g almond flour

Pinch of salt

100g powdered sugar alternative

3 medium lemons

3 large eggs

Method:

1. Mix butter, 100g almond flour, 25g of the sugar substitute and a pinch of salt into a bowl

2. Press mixture into an 8×8" lined baking dish

3. Bake for 20 minutes at 175°C

4. Cool for 10 minutes

5. Zest one of the lemons into a bowl

6. Juice all of the lemons and then add into the bowl with the eggs, the remaining sugar substitute, the remaining almond flour and the salt

7. Stir well to combine

8. Pour the filling onto the crust and bake for 25 mins

9. Take out and allow to cool. Sprinkle a little bit more sugar substitute on top and enjoy

Snack Ideas

Celery Sticks with Unsweetened Peanut Butter: Serves 1

Prep time/ Cook time:

5 mins

Ingredients:

1-2 celery sticks

(trimmed and halved)

Crunchy or smooth unsweetened peanut butter

Method:

Spread each celery stick with the peanut butter and enjoy!

Almond Crackers: Serves 6

Prep time/ Cook time:

10 mins/ 10-15 mins

Ingredients:

190g almond flour (can use ground almonds but texture will differ)

½ tsp sea salt

1 large egg

Method:

1. Preheat the oven to 180°C and line a baking sheet with parchment paper

2. Mix the almond flour and sea salt in a large bowl. Add the egg and mix well, until a dough forms. You could also use a food processor

3. Place the dough between two large pieces of parchment paper. Use a rolling pin to roll out into a rectangle, about 2 cm thick. If it rolls into an oval shape just rip off pieces of dough and re-attach to form a more rectangular shape

4. Cut the cracker dough into rectangles. Prick with a fork or toothpick to prevent it from bubbling

5. Place on the lined baking sheet and bake for 10-12 minutes until golden

Garlic and Coriander Olives: Makes 4 Portions

Prep time/ Cook time:

5 mins

Ingredients:

1 tbsp coriander (chopped)

1 small jar green pitted olives

2-3 garlic cloves, chopped

Method:

1. Mix all ingredients together

These can be stored in an airtight container in the fridge for up to a week

Hard Boiled Eggs

Prep time/ Cook time:
8 mins

Ingredients:
Eggs
I often take a few out with me in case I can't find somewhere that can do low carb food, or I just want a quick snack. You can also cut them in half vertically and put fillings in such as bacon, lettuce and tomato with mayonnaise for an egg BLT!

Method:
Bring a saucepan of water to a boil. Add eggs and cook for 8 minutes

Keto Sausage Rolls: Makes 10

Prep time/ Cook time:
15 mins/ 25- 30 mins

Ingredients:

For the pastry:
450g mozzarella cheese, shredded
3 tbsp full fat cream cheese

3 eggs (beat 2 together and beat 1 on its own separately)

49g almond flour

30g coconut flour

1 tsp baking powder

½ tsp xanthan gum

For the sausage filling:

1 lb / 300g sausage meat (if using sausages, take off the skins)

85g pork rinds / pork scratchings, crushed

25g finely chopped celery

13g white onion, minced / very finely chopped

1 tsp garlic powder

½ tsp / pinch of salt

½ tsp pepper

My son now prefers these to ordinary sausage rolls!

Method:

1. Preheat oven to 200°C (190°C for fan oven) 400°F. Melt the shredded mozzarella and the cream cheese in a frying pan over medium heat. (This step can also be done in a microwave) Remove from the heat, then stir the melted cheeses until they're well combined. Using a mixing bowl, add the almond flour, coconut flour, baking powder, Xanthan gum and 2 of the eggs to the cheese mixture. Mix until well combined.

2. In a large bowl, mix the raw sausage (removed from the casings) with the minced onion and celery. Add the crushed pork rinds, onion and garlic powder and salt and pepper. Mix thoroughly.

3. Cut some baking parchment 20 inches long and along one side, spread the pastry into a long tube. Fold the parchment paper over the mixture and using your hands or a rolling pin, press the mixture into a flat rectangle wide enough to roll around the sausage meat

4. Spread the sausage meat evenly along one side of the pastry mixture leaving a gap to seal it. Brush the edge with the remaining beaten egg

5. Use the parchment to roll the pastry mixture over (a bit like a swiss roll) over the sausage meat. Press together gently until sealed

6. Divide the long sausage roll into 10 with a sharp knife. Place the sausage rolls seal down on a parchment paper lined baking tray. (This was when I patched up the seal on some of them too!)

7. Brush generously with the egg. Bake for 25-30 mins. I turned the, round halfway as the outsides browned quicker. 10. Once evenly browned, use a fresh sheet of parchment or use a very non stick tray and turn on the side to crisp up the bottom

Avocado Crisps: Makes 15

Prep time/ Cook time:

5 mins/40 mins

Ingredients:

1 avocado

35g freshly grated Parmesan

1 tsp lemon juice

1/2 tsp. garlic powder

1/2 tsp Italian seasoning

Salt

Freshly ground black pepper

Method:

1. Preheat oven to 160°C and line two baking sheets with parchment paper

2. In a medium bowl, mash avocado with a fork until smooth. Stir in Parmesan, lemon juice, garlic powder, and Italian seasoning. Season with salt and pepper

3. Place heaped teaspoon-size scoops of mixture onto a baking sheet, leaving about 3 inches gap between each scoop

4. Flatten each scoop to 3 inches wide across with the back of a spoon or measuring cup

5. Bake for about 30 minutes until crisp and golden, then let cool completely. Serve at room temperature

Kale Crisps: Serves 2-3

Prep time/ Cook time:
5 mins/10-15 mins

Ingredients:
450g kale
1 tbsp olive oil
½ tsp white wine vinegar
salt

Method:
1. Preheat the oven to 150°C
2. Rinse the kale and tear into smaller pieces
3. Toss the kale ien olive oil and lemon juice or white wine vinegar and sprinkle on salt
4. Pop the kale onto a lined baking sheet and bake in the oven for 10-15 minutes, until the kale is crispy

Halloumi And Bacon Bites: Serves 2

Prep time/ Cook time:
5 mins/10-15 mins

Ingredients:
250g halloumi
6 rashers of streaky bacon

Method:

1. Preheat your oven to 200°C

2. Cut your halloumi lengthways into strips

3. Wrap a piece of bacon around the halloumi so it's completely encased

4. Pop into the oven on a lined baking sheet for 10-15 mins, turning halfway

Charcuterie Platter: Serves 1-2

Prep time/ Cook time:

15 mins

Ingredients:

50g blue cheese

50g cheddar

50g halloumi

Parma ham

Salami or chorizo

Proscuitto

Gherkins (sugar free)

Cherry tomatoes

Olives- black and green

Cashew nuts

Pistachios

Salsa

Method:

1. Assemble your choice of charcuterie and cheese onto a big wooden board

2. Decorate with the gherkins, tomatoes and olives and anything else keto friendly that you fancy. The items in the ingredients section are just suggestions!

Mini Frittatas: Serves 6

Prep time/ Cook time:

5 mins / 15-20 mins

Ingredients:

6 eggs

salt

pepper

A big handful of spinach

2 mushrooms

A handful of cherry tomatoes

25g cheddar cheese

Method:

1. Break the eggs into a bowl, season and whisk

2. Preheat an oven to 180°C

3. Grease a muffin tin

4. Pour egg mixture into the muffin tins, dividing the mixture equally

5. Pop whatever toppings you fancy on top of the egg mixture

6. Bake for 15-20 mins until set

The Mediterranean Diet

The Mediterranean diet is a nice alternative to keto to combine with fasting. Let's remind ourselves how the plan works. As we discussed in previous chapters, the Mediterranean diet is in general, less restrictive than the keto diet. It focuses on the foods of the countries in the Mediterranean region.

The focuses of these country's diets are:

- Fresh fruit- Apples, bananas, oranges, peaches, figs, melon, pears, grapes and berries
- Vegetables- Tomatoes, broccoli, kale, spinach, cucumbers, potatoes, sweet potatoes, carrots
- Wholegrains- Wholegrain pasta, wild rice, wholegrain bread
- Nuts and seeds- Almonds, hazelnuts, cashews, chia seeds, pumpkin seeds and sunflower seeds
- Legumes- Beans, chickpeas, lentils and kidney beans
- Seafood- Fish and shellfish such as salmon, mussels, lobster, trout, mackerel and swordfish
- Eggs
- Poultry- Chicken, turkey and duck
- Olive oil and other healthy fats such as avocado oil

The diet also includes a small amount of alcohol, dairy and red meat, in moderation. Although the focus is on fresh, you can still benefit from eating frozen and tinned vegetables.

What foods should you limit/avoid?

- Sugar- ice cream, fizzy drinks, cakes and chocolate. Try and get your sweet fix from yoghurt and fruit. A small amount of dark chocolate is another option if you are having sweet cravings
- Processed meat- burgers, sausage, reformed meat, bacon, anything breaded or glazed. Some charcuterie meat such as parma ham is fine though
- Fast food- avoid anything deep fried in unhealthy oil, like fries
- Refined grains- white bread, white rice, white pasta, crisps
- Microwave meals- most of these are packed with sugars and additives
- Unhealthy fats- trans fats, saturated fats

As with the keto recipes before, here is a variety of Mediterranean recipes, to suit each mealtime.

Breakfasts

Avocado On Wholegrain Toast With Egg: Serves 1

Prep time/ Cook time:
5 mins 5 mins

Ingredients:
½ avocado
1 egg
1 slice of wholegrain bread
lime
salt and pepper
chilli flakes

Method:
1. Mash the avocado into a bowl and add lime juice and salt and pepper to taste
2. Put tbsp of olive oil into a pan and gently warm.
3. Crack your egg into pan and fry slowly with the lid on so that it cooks gently and steams
4. Toast your wholegrain bread and spread it liberally with the mashed avocado
5. Top with your fried egg and for an extra kick, sprinkle with chilli flakes

Spinach And Parmesan Cakes: Serves 2

Prep time/ Cook time:

10 mins / 20 mins

Ingredients:

340g fresh spinach

80g cottage cheese

45g parmesan cheese, plus more for garnish

2 large eggs, beaten

1 clove garlic, minced

¼ teaspoon salt

¼ teaspoon freshly ground pepper

Method:

1. Preheat the oven to 200°C

2. Use a food processor to blitz spinach. Pop into a mixing bowl

3. Add the cottage cheese, parmesan, garlic, eggs and seasoning and stir

4. Spray an 8 hole muffin pan with spray oil and divide up the mixture between the muffin tray

5. Bake for 20 mins until set

Serve warm from the oven with more parmesan to garnish

Spanish Omelette: Serves 4

Prep time/ Cook time:

10 mins/ 50 mins

Ingredients:

500g new potatoes

1 onion

150ml olive oil

6 eggs

3 tbsp flat-leaf parsley

Method:

1. Chop the potatoes into thick slices and chop the onion

2. Heat the oil in a big frying pan, add the potatoes and onion and cook on low heat for 30 mins, stirring occasionally

3. Strain the potatoes and onion through a colander and keep the oil aside

4. Beat the eggs in a separate bowl, then stir into the potatoes with the parsley and salt and pepper

5. Heat some of the oil in a pan and tip everything in, using a spatula to form the shape of the mixture

6. When nearly set, turn over on a plate and then slide back onto the pan and cook for a little bit longer

7. Turn over twice more and then serve

Blueberry Smoothie: Serves 1

Prep time/ Cook time:
5 mins/2 mins

Ingredients:
75g blueberries
2 small ripe bananas
400ml semi-skimmed milk
½ tsp vanilla extract

Method:
1. Peel and slice the bananas
2. Pop the blueberries and the bananas into a blender
3. Add the milk and the vanilla
4. Blend and pour into a chilled glass and enjoy!

Shakshuka Eggs: Serves 4-6

Prep time/ Cook time:
10 mins/25 mins

Ingredients:
3 tbsp olive oil
1 onion, halved and thinly sliced
1 red pepper, seeded and thinly sliced
3 garlic cloves, thinly sliced

1 tsp ground cumin

1 tsp paprika

1/8 tsp ground cayenne pepper

1 tin plum tomatoes with their juices, chopped up roughly

¾ tsp salt

¼ tsp black pepper

140g feta, crumbled

6 large eggs

Chopped coriander

Method:

1. Heat oven to 190°C
2. Heat oil in a large pan and set the heat to medium
3. Add sliced onion and red pepper. Cook until soft, for about 20 mins
4. Add garlic and cook for 1 to 2 minutes
5. Stir in the spices and cook for a further minute
6. Add the tomatoes and season with salt and pepper. Leave to simmer for about 10 minutes.
7. Season and stir in the feta cheese
8. Crack the eggs into the pans over the tomatoes.
9. Transfer the pan to the oven and bake the eggs until set, for about 10 mins
10. Garnish with coriander

Mackerel With Spinach Eggs: Serves 4

Prep time/ Cook time:
15 mins / 15 mins

Ingredients:
200g spinach
3 tbsp crème fraîche
3 tbsp snipped fresh chives
200g smoked mackerel, skin removed
8 medium free-range eggs
Lemon wedges to serve

Method:
1. Heat your oven to 200°C
2. Wilt your spinach by putting the spinach into a bowl and pour it over hot water
3. Use a sieve or colander to drain the spinach of water
4. Mix the crème fraiche with the chives and season
5. Divide the spinach between individual ovenproof dishes (I used large ramekin style dishes)
6. Divide the mackerel between, then share out the crème fraîche mixture
7. Crack 2 eggs into each dish. Season with salt and pepper
8. Cover each dish with foil and bake for 15 mins until the eggs are set

9. Serve with lemon wedges

Spinach, Wholemeal Wrap with Eggs and Feta: Serves 1

Prep time/ Cook time:
10 mins/5 mins

Ingredients:
1 wholewheat tortilla
1 ½ tsp coconut oil
handful of baby spinach leaves
1 sundried tomato
2 eggs
25g feta cheese
1 tomato- diced

Method:
1. Melt coconut oil in a pan over medium heat
2. Saute spinach and tomato in the pan until the spinach wilts
3. Add eggs and scramble, sprinkle feta cheese over the eggs and cook until the cheese melts
4. Warm the tortilla in a separate pan
5. Pop the egg mixture onto the tortilla and top the diced tomato
6. Roll tortilla and place back into the pan to set it

Mango and Pineapple Overnight Oats: Serves 1

Prep time/ Cook time:

10 mins/ 8 hrs

Ingredients:

52g pineapple

1 tbsp dried mango

175ml coconut milk

1 ½ tsp chia seeds

50g oats

Method:

1. Combine all of the ingredients into a kilner style jar or a bowl and refrigerate overnight

Greek Pancakes: Makes 4

Prep time/ Cook time:

10 mins/ 5 mins

Ingredients:

2 eggs

150g Greek yoghurt

1 tsp baking powder

60ml milk

95g wholewheat flour

1 tsp olive oil

Method:

1. Mix the eggs and milk together and whisk
2. Add the Greek yoghurt and whisk until there are no remaining lumps
3. Mix the flour and the baking powder in a separate bowl
4. Combine the two mixtures together
5. Add the olive oil to a pan and pour a small amount of batter onto the pan
6. Cook for 2 mins on either side until golden

Serve with fruit and honey.

Sweet Potato Breakfast Hash: Serves 4

Prep time/ Cook time:

15 mins / 35 mins

Ingredients:

2 sweet potatoes

3 tbsp olive oil divided

1 tsp smoked paprika

½ tsp salt

½ tsp pepper

2 onions, chopped

2 sausages (already cooked and sliced)

1 red pepper, chopped

6 portobello mushrooms, sliced

1 tbsp balsamic vinegar

8 eggs

Method:

1. Set your oven to 200°C

2. Peel and cut your potatoes into 2 cm size pieces

3. Spread the potatoes onto a lined baking sheet.

5. Add 2 tbsp of olive oil, paprika and salt and pepper and cover the potatoes fully

6. Bake for 10 mins

7. Remove the potatoes from the oven and add the onions, sausages, mushrooms and pepper. Drizzle another tbsp of olive oil and a tbsp of balsamic vinegar onto the mix. Mix well

8. Bake for another 20 mins, then remove from the oven

9. Crack the eggs into the pan and cook for another 5-7 mins

Lunches

Bulgar Wheat Salad: Serves 4

Prep time/ Cook time:

15 mins/5mins

Ingredients:

250g bulgar wheat

15g flat leaf parsley, chopped

10g chives, chopped

15g mint leaves, chopped

1 cucumber, diced

1 red onion, chopped

200g cherry tomatoes, halved

100g radishes, thinly sliced

100ml olive oil

3 tbsp balsamic vinegar

1 tsp Dijon mustard

1 clove garlic, finely chopped

1 tsp runny honey

Method:

1. Set a large pan of water to boil

2. Add the bulgar wheat and simmer for 10-15 mins

3. Drain and cool the bulgar

4. In a bowl, whisk together the dijon mustard, balsamic, garlic, olive oil and honey together

5. Mix the rest of the ingredients in with the bulgar and drizzle the dressing over the top

Halloumi and Watermelon Salad: Makes 4 Servings

Prep time/ Cook time:

5 mins/ 10 mins

Ingredients:

½ a watermelon

250g halloumi

4 tbsp olive oil

15 kalamata olives

mint leaves to serve

2 tbsp balsamic vinegar

Method:

1. Slice the watermelon into cubes and place on a large serving platter

2. Heat 2 tbsp of the olive oil into a pan and fry the halloumi in strips until golden

3. Combine the remaining olive oil and balsamic

4. Pop the halloumi, olives and mint leaves on top of the melon and drizzle the dressing on top

Fig and Goat's Cheese Salad: Serves 1

Prep time/ Cook time:

10 mins

Ingredients:

Large handful of mixed salad leaves

4 dried figs, chopped

30g goat's cheese

2 tsp olive oil

2 tsp balsamic vinegar

½ tsp honey

Pinch of salt

Black pepper

Method:

1. Stir together the oil, vinegar, honey and salt and pepper to make the dressing

2. Mix the salad leaves, figs and goat's cheese in a separate bowl

3. Pour over the dressing and toss well

Mediterranean Baked Cod: Serves 4

Prep time/ Cook time:

15 mins/ 15 mins

Ingredients:

4 cod fillets

½ tsp salt

115ml lemon juice

1 tbsp Dijon mustard

2 onions, sliced thin

2 tomatoes, diced

2 garlic cloves, minced

35g capers drained

½ tsp pepper

2 tbsp rosemary, dried or fresh

60ml olive oil

Method:

1. Preheat oven to 175°C
2. Sprinkle salt on cod fillets
3. Whisk together lemon juice and mustard in a small bowl
4. Cut baking paper into a large rectangle, enough that the fish can fit and a 'tent' can be made with the paper
5. Put a small amount of onions on the parcel, then pop one of the cod fillets on top. Do this for each piece of fish

6. Add onions, capers, pepper, rosemary and diced tomatoes on top of the fish

7. Divide the lemon and mustard mix between each fish and pop some olive oil on top

8. Scrunch the baking paper together to make a 'tent'

9. Bake for 15 mins

Spaghetti Alle Vongole: Serves 2

Prep time/ Cook time:

15 mins / 12 mins

Ingredients:

140g spaghetti

500g fresh clams in shells

2 large tomatoes

olive oil

1 garlic clove chopped

1 small red chill, finely chopped

60 ml white wine

handful of chopped parsley

Method:

1. Set a large pan of salted water on the heat for the spaghetti

2. Rinse the clams several times in several changes of cold water

3. Get rid of any that are open or damaged

4. Cover the tomatoes with boiling water, leave for 1 min then remove their skins

5. Cook the spaghetti

6. Heat the oil in a pan, add the chili and garlic and fry for a minute

7. Stir in the tomatoes, add the clams and the wine and bring to a boil

8. Season well and cook for 4-5 mins until the clams open up

9. Drain the pasta and tip into the pan of sauce. Garnish with parsley and serve

Greek Lemon Chicken Soup: Makes 6 Servings

Prep time/ Cook time:
10 mins/20 mins

Ingredients:
2 tbsp olive oil
450g boneless, skinless chicken thighs, cut into 1-inch chunks
salt and black pepper
4 cloves garlic, minced
1 onion, chopped
3 carrots, sliced

2 celery stalks, cut in half lengthways and sliced

½ tsp dried thyme

2 litres chicken stock

2 bay leaves

850g cannellini beans

900g spinach

2 tbsp fresh lemon juice

2 tbsp fresh parsley

2 tbsp fresh dill

Method:

1. Heat 1 tbsp of oil in a large pot

2. Season the chicken and cook until golden, for about 5 mins. Take the chicken out and set aside

3. Add the last of the oil to the pot. Add the garlic, onion, carrot and celery. Cook until tender

4. Stir in the thyme and cook for 1 min

5. Whisk in the chicken stock and bay leaves and bring to a boil

6. Reduce the heat and stir in the cannellini beans and the chicken

7. Cook until the sauce has thickened and the chicken is cooked, this should take about 15 mins

8. Stir in the spinach, lemon juice, parsley and dill and season well. Cook for another 2 mins and serve

Caprese Salad: Serves 4

Prep time/ Cook time:

20 mins

Ingredients:

1 tbsp olive oil

1 tbsp balsamic vinegar

1 tsp Dijon mustard

2 tomatoes

225g mozzarella

9 basil leaves

¼ teaspoon sea salt

¼ tsp black pepper

Method:

1. Whisk the mustard, balsamic and olive oil together until they are nicely combined

2. Slice the tomatoes into thin rounds

3. Slice the mozzarella into rounds

4. Arrange the tomato and mozzarella alternately on a large plate

5. Scatter the basil evenly over the plate

6. Season the plate and drizzle with the dressing

Picnic Pasta Salad: Serves 3

Prep time/ Cook time:

5 mins / 15 mins

Ingredients:

300g uncooked small shaped pasta

200g feta cheese

250g cherry tomatoes

1 orange pepper, diced

60g rocket

bunch of spring onions

Bunch of basil leaves

Handful of chopped mint

Handful of chopped parsley

1 tbsp dijon mustard

3 tbsp lemon juice

60ml olive oil

3 garlic cloves, minced

1 tsp Italian seasoning

½ tsp salt

Method:

1. Cook the pasta according to the instructions
2. Whizz together the mustard, lemon juice, olive oil, minced garlic, Italian seasoning and salt to make the dressing

3. Chop the feta cheese into small pieces

4. Chop the peppers, spring onions and herbs

5. Drain the pasta and pop into a big bowl together with the vegetables and herbs

6. Mix the dressing in with the pasta and mix well

Chicken Quinoa Bowl: Serves 4

Prep time/ Cook time:

5 mins 30 mins

Ingredients:

450g skinless, boneless chicken breasts sliced thinly

4 tbsp olive oil

3 tbsp butter

5-6 large garlic cloves, minced

½ small red onion, chopped

60ml cup lemon juice

360g quinoa

475ml water

50g rocket

12 cherry tomatoes

salt and black pepper to taste

Method:

1. Rinse the quinoa in cold water and add to a saucepan. Add the rinsed quinoa, pop the lid on and simmer for 20 mins

2. Remove from the heat and set aside, fluff with a fork

3. Melt 2 tbsp of the butter with 3 tbsp oil in a large pan

4. Add chicken and garlic and cook for 3 mins. Give everything a good mix and cook for another 3 mins

5. Heat the remaining oil in a separate pan, add the tomatoes and onion and cook until soft

6. Remove them to a bowl and pour lemon juice into the pan you've just used

7. As soon as the lemon juice is warm, add the remaining butter and stir until melted

8. Add the cooked chicken and the tomato and onion mixture back into the lemon mix. Spoon the quinoa in and mix well

9. Remove the pan from the heat and add the rocket. Season well and serve

Harissa Chickpea Grain Bowl: Serves 2

Prep time/ Cook time:
10 mins/45 mins

Ingredients:
1 large aubergine
Salt and black pepper
1 onion, diced
3 garlic cloves, minced
400g tomato puree
400g chickpeas
2 tbsp harissa paste
175g millet grain
475ml water
2 tbsp avocado oil
Coriander to garnish

Method:
1. Add the water to a pan and add the millet. Cook for 25 mins until the millet is cooked, then set aside
2. Heat 1 tbsp of the oil in a large pan. Dice the aubergine, season it and add to the pan. Cook for about ten mins
3. Remove the aubergine to a bowl and heat the remaining oil in a pan
4. Add the onion and cook gently for about ten mins

5. Add the garlic and cook for 2 mins

6. Add the chickpeas, harissa and tomato

7. Pop the aubergine back in the pan and simmer for 15 mins

8. Divide the millet into two bowls, top with the aubergine mixture and garnish with coriander

Dinners

<u>Mediterranean Fish Stew: Serves 3</u>

Prep time/ Cook time:
5 mins/25 mins

Ingredients:
2 tbsp butter
2 tbsp olive oil
1 onion, chopped
1 carrot, sliced into thin rounds
1 tbsp flour
3 medium potatoes, peeled and cut into bite sized cubes
450g white fish
950ml chicken broth
½ tsp smoked paprika
Salt and pepper, to taste

Method:
1. Heat the butter and the oil in a big saucepan

214

2. Add carrots and onions and sauté until soft

3. Stir in flour and then add potatoes, cook for 1 minute

4. Add chicken stock and bring to a boil

5. Add fish and the paprika then cover and simmer, stirring occasionally for about 20 mins

Lamb Stew with Spinach: Serves 4

Prep time/ Cook time:

15 mins/1hr 15 mins

Ingredients:

450g diced lamb shoulder

2 garlic cloves, crushed

60ml olive oil

1 large onion, chopped

2 carrots, sliced

425 g chickpeas

100g tomato puree

125ml liquid chicken stock

2 tbsp fresh lemon juice

salt and pepper

285g spinach, stems removed and chopped

Method:

1. Sprinkle salt, pepper and garlic onto the lamb

2. Heat oil in a large pot. Add the lamb and sauté for 10 mins

3. Add onion and carrots and sauté until beginning to brown, about 5 minutes

4. Add chickpeas, chicken stock, tomato puree and lemon juice and bring to a boil

5. Reduce the heat and simmer for an hour

6. Add spinach to stew, cook until the spinach wilts

7. Season with salt and pepper

Morrocan Chickpea and Chicken: Serves 4

Prep time/ Cook time:

40 mins / 30 mins

Ingredients:

4 chicken breasts

2 red peppers

1 yellow pepper

1 medium red onion

2 medium courgettes

1 tbsp olive oil

½tsp dried crushed chillies

400g chickpeas, drained and rinsed

150ml low fat natural yogurt

fresh flat leaf parsley or coriander, to garnish (optional)

2 garlic cloves, peeled and crushed

2 tsp ground cumin

2 tsp ground coriander

216

1 tsp harissa paste

juice of ½ lemon

sea salt

freshly ground black pepper

Method:

1. Mix the garlic, coriander, cumin, harissa, lemon juice, salt and pepper to make a marinade

2. Make a couple of slashes in each chicken breast, pop in a bowl and add the marinade

3. Cover and chill for 30 mins

4. Preheat the oven to 200°C and line a baking tray

5. Pop the chicken onto the tray, slashed side up and bake for 25 mins until the juices run clear

6. In the meantime, cut the onion into wedges and chop the peppers and courgettes

7. Mix the olive oil, chillies and salt and pepper together and toss the vegetables in it

8. Stir-fry the vegetables in a large frying pan for 6-8 mins until tender

9. Add the chickpeas and cook for a further 2 mins

10. Top the chicken breasts with the vegetable mixture and serve with the yoghurt

Garlic and Thyme Salmon: Serves 4

Prep time/ Cook time:

5 mins / 40 mins

Ingredients:

1kg potatoes

4 tbsp olive oil

2 garlic cloves, finely sliced

Fresh thyme sprigs

4 large salmon fillets

Finely grated zest and juice of 1 lemon

2 tbsp capers, rinsed

400g cherry tomatoes

200ml dry white wine

Method:

1. Preheat the oven to 200°C

2. Peel and chop the potatoes into thick slices. Pop them into a pan and parboil the slices for 4 mins

3. Take a large oven dish and pour in 1 tbsp of oil. Empty the potatoes, thyme and garlic into the dish and season

4. Bake for 20 minutes

5. Sear the salmon for 2 mins on either side

6. When the 20 mins is up, put the fish in with the potatoes, add the lemon juice and zest

7. Add the capers, tomatoes and wine and bake for 15 mins until the fish and potatoes are cooked

Seafood Paella: Serves 4

Prep time/ Cook time:
20 mins / 30 mins

Ingredients:
175g raw tiger prawns
150g mussels, cleaned and de-bearded
150g raw squid rings
1 onion
3 garlic cloves, crushed
1 tsp paprika
250g paella rice
900ml fish stock
pinch saffron
1 ½ tbsp extra-virgin olive oil
30g flat leaf parsley
1 tsp paprika
285g roasted peppers
230g chopped tomatoes
1 lemon, cut into wedges

Method:

1.Heat the oil in a big frying pan and fry the chopped onion for 5 mins until soft

2. Add crushed garlic cloves, chopped tomatoes, half of the parsley and paprika fry for 2 minutes

3. Stir in the paella rice and season well

4. Add saffron to the stock, pour the stock into the pan and bring to a boil

5. Reduce to a simmer and leave the rice to cook without stirring for 10 minutes

6. Put in the roasted peppers and cook for another minute

7. Add in the raw black tiger prawns, mussels and raw squid rings. Cook for a further 5 minutes

8. Take off the heat, cover with foil and rest for 5 mins

Serve with lemon wedges and the rest of the parsley

Feta Stuffed Chicken Breast: Serves 4

Prep time/ Cook time:

10 mins/35 mins

Ingredients:

115g feta cheese, cubed

1 small red pepper, deseeded and chopped

114 spinach

45g olives

1 tbsp fresh basil

1 tbsp flat-leaf parsley, chopped

2 cloves garlic, minced

4 chicken breasts

¼ teaspoon salt

½ teaspoon ground pepper

1 tbsp olive oil

1 tbsp lemon juice

Method:

1. Preheat oven to 200°C

2. Mix the feta, red pepper, spinach, olives, basil, parsley and garlic in a bowl

3. Cut a slice into each chicken breast to form a pocket

4. Stuff the chicken with the mixture, distributing between them. Secure them shut with wooden picks

5. Season the chicken

6. Line a baking tray and pop the chicken into the oven. Bake for 25-35 mins until the chicken is cooked

7. Remove the picks before serving and sprinkle liberally with lemon juice

Broccoli and Lemon Pasta: Serves 2

Prep time/ Cook time:

10 mins/20 mins

Ingredients:

200g wholemeal penne

1 leek, sliced thinly

200g broccoli, cut into small florets

1 tbsp olive oil

1 red pepper, deseeded and chopped

1 tsp fresh chopped rosemary

1 red chilli deseeded and sliced

3 sliced garlic cloves

1 lemon (zested and juiced)

3 tbsp ricotta

Method:

1. Boil the pasta with the leeks for 7 mins, then add the broccoli and boil for 5 mins more until just tender

2. In a large pan, heat the oil and fry the pepper with the chilli, garlic and rosemary for 5 mins

3. Drain the pasta and vegetables, keeping back some of the pasta water

4. Combine the pasta and the vegetables, add the lemon zest and juice, ricotta and a little of the pasta water

5. Serve in bowls for maximum comfort value!

Pork Stifado: Serves 4

Prep time/ Cook time:

25 mins/ 1hr 45 mins

Ingredients:

20 small pickling onions

750g pork steaks

8 garlic cloves

1 bay leaf

Rosemary sprig

2 thyme sprigs

3 tbsp olive oil

350ml red wine

500ml passata

1 tbsp tomato puree

3 tbsp red wine vinegar

2 tbsp currants

salt and pepper

Method:

1. Pop the unpeeled onions into the water and boil them for 2 mins

2. Drain them, let them cool and peel them

3. Cut the pork into cubes. Peel the garlic and leave them whole

4. Heat the oil in a pan and brown it, transferring it to a plate when seared

5. Drain the pan of any excess oil. Pop back the meat into the pan, add the garlic and red wine and let cook for a couple of mins

6. Add the passata, tomato, red wine vinegar and herbs

7. Add the onions, reduce the heat and simmer for 45 mins

8. Add the currants and simmer for another 45 mins

9. Season and serve

Prawns with New Potatoes and Peas: Serves 2

Prep time/ Cook time:

15 mins/ 20 mins

Ingredients:

400g new potatoes

3 fennel bulbs

200g peas

140g raw prawns- de-veined

1 tsp tarragon

2 tbsp flat leaf parsley

1 lemon

50g feta

Method:

1. Pop the potatoes into a pan and just cover them with salted water

2. Boil for 5 mins. After 5 mins slice the fennel and add to the water

3. Boil for another 5 mins then add the peas

4. The water should have cooked down by this point, so add the prawns and tarragon, stir them until they turn pink

5. Add the parsley, the feta and the lemon juice and serve immediately

Baked sea bass: Serves 2

Prep time/ Cook time:

10 mins/35 mins

Ingredients:

450g sea bass (cleaned and scaled

3 garlic cloves, minced

1 tbsp olive oil

1 tbsp Italian seasoning

2 tsp black pepper

1 tsp salt

2 lemon wedges

78ml white wine

Method:

1. Preheat oven to 230°C

2. Mix the garlic, olive oil, salt, and black pepper

3. Place the fish into a baking dish with high sides

4. Rub the fish with the garlic and oil mixture

5. Pour the wine over the fish, bake for 15 mins

6. Add parsley and Italian seasoning and cook for a further 5 mins

7. Plate and drizzle the juices over the fish. Garnish with lemon wedges

Side Dishes

Mixed Bean Salad: Serves 3-4

Prep time/ Cook time:

10 mins

Ingredients:

425g cannellini beans

425g black beans

425g chickpeas

300g sweetcorn

1 red pepper-diced

½ red onion- diced

1 tomato- diced

1 garlic clove, minced

Handful of coriander

1 tsp apple cider vinegar

1 lime, juiced

1 tsp olive oil

1 tsp cumin

1 tsp ground coriander

Salt and pepper

Method:

1. Mix all of the wet ingredients together in a large mixing bowl

2. Add the beans, diced vegetables and herbs and mix well

3. Leave to chill and serve

Patatas Bravas: Serves 4

Prep time/ Cook time:

10 mins/35 mins

Ingredients:

POTATOES

675-900 g red skin potatoes, quartered into bite size pieces

2-3 tbsp olive oil

½ tsp sea salt

½ tsp garlic powder

SAUCE

1 tbsp olive oil

1/2 white or yellow onion, diced

3 cloves garlic, minced

1/2 tsp sea salt

1/2 tsp paprika

1 pinch cayenne or red pepper flake

1 tsp garlic powder

170g tomato passata

1-2 tsp hot sauce

360 ml water

Method:

1. Soak quartered potatoes in very hot water for 10-15 minutes. In the meantime, preheat oven to 230°C

2. Once potatoes are soaked, dry thoroughly and then add to a baking sheet. Sprinkle with olive oil, sea salt and garlic powder. Toss to coat

3. Bake for 20-25 minutes or until golden brown and cooked through, stirring once

4. While the potatoes are baking, heat 1 tbsp olive oil in a large skillet over medium-low heat. Add onion and garlic and salt and stir. Cook for 7-8 minutes until the mixture becomes translucent and very fragrant. If it begins to brown, turn down the heat to low and stir frequently

5. Add paprika, garlic powder, cayenne and stir. Then add passata, hot sauce and water and stir

6. Cook for 10-12 minutes or until simmering and the flavours are well blended. Reduce heat if it begins to bubble too vigorously. Taste and adjust seasonings as needed. For a smooth sauce, puree in a small blender or food processor until smooth

7. Remove potatoes from the oven and sprinkle with a bit more salt and garlic to taste. Place in a serving dishes and drizzle with tomato sauce

Spanakorizo (Greek Rice): Serves 2

Prep time/ Cook time:
5 mins/40 mins

Ingredients:
1kg fresh or frozen spinach, rinsed and stemmed
200g brown rice
118ml olive oil
4 spring onions, chopped
1 red onion, finely chopped
1 leek, sliced
½ bunch dill, finely chopped
150g tinned chopped tomatoes
1 tbsp tomato paste
1 cube vegetable stock
salt and freshly ground pepper
½ a lemon, juiced

60g feta cheese

Method:

1. Heat the olive oil over medium heat. Add the onions, spring onions and leek and sauté for 3-4 minutes, until translucent

2. Add the spinach and stir for a few minutes, until wilted. Stir in the tomatoes, the tomato paste, two cups of hot water, the vegetable stock, the rice and season

3. Reduce heat to low and simmer, covered, for about 30 mins until the rice is cooked

4. Add more water if necessary

5. Season with salt and pepper to taste

6. Garnish with dill, lemon juice and feta cheese

Balsamic Roasted Vegetables: Serves 5

Prep time/ Cook time:

10 mins / 40 mins

Ingredients:

1 large sweet potato

2 carrots

2 large flat mushrooms, cubed

1 large red onion

2 cloves garlic, sliced

2 tbsp balsamic vinegar

4 tbsp olive oil

1 aubergine

1 tsp fresh thyme

1 tsp rosemary

1 tsp chopped sage

½ tsp salt

½ black pepper

Method:

1. Preheat oven to 200°C and lightly oil a large roasting pan

2. Chop the sweet potato, onion and carrots into 2-inch pieces

3. Mix them with the oil, balsamic, garlic and herbs

4. Roast for 15 mins, then add the aubergine

5. Roast for another 15 mins then add the mushrooms

6. Cook for a further 10 mins

7. Season and serve

<u>Mediterranean Couscous: Serves 2-3</u>

Prep time/ Cook time:

5 mins/5 mins

Ingredients:

200g couscous

1 vegetable stock cube

250g cherry tomatoes halved

2 avocados, peeled, stoned and chopped

150g pack mozzarella, drained and chopped

A handful rocket

1 heaped tbsp pesto

1 tbsp lemon juice

3 tbsp olive oil

Method:

1. Mix the couscous and stock in a bowl, pour over 300ml boiling water, then cover with a plate and leave for 5 mins

2. Mix the pesto with the lemon juice and some seasoning, then gradually mix in the oil. Pour over the couscous and mix with a fork

3. Mix the tomatoes, avocado and mozzarella into the couscous, then lightly stir in the rocket

<u>Lemon and Garlic Asparagus: Serves 2-3</u>

Prep time/ Cook time:

5 mins/15 mins

Ingredients:

1 bunch asparagus

60 ml olive oil

2 tbsp water

½ lemon, juiced

½ lemon, cut into wedges

4 cloves garlic, minced

Salt and black pepper

Method:

1. Heat the oil and the water in a frying pan, add the asparagus and stir until it's all coated

2. Bring to a boil, add salt and pepper

3. Simmer for 2 mins

4. Add the garlic and lemon juice

5. Cook until the asparagus is tender but crisp

6. Serve with the lemon wedges

<u>Crispy Polenta with Cherry Tomatoes: Serves 2</u>

Prep time/ Cook time:

2 hrs 5 mins/30 mins

Ingredients:

340g cherry tomatoes

Salt and pepper

3 ¼ tbsp olive oil

230g quick cook polenta

1 litre of water

4 sprigs of thyme

56g goat cheese

Method:

1. Oil a dish for the polenta
2. In a large saucepan, bring the water and the olive oil to the boil
3. Whisk in the polenta. Cook over low heat, whisking, until thick for about 5 minutes
4. Season with salt and black pepper to taste
5. Transfer the polenta to the prepared baking dish and smooth the top. Chill for 2 hours until firm
6. Preheat the oven to 180°C and line a deep baking tray
7. Mix the tomatoes with 1 ¼ tbsp of olive oil and season
8. Pop them onto the baking sheet and add the thyme
9. Roast for 20 mins, removing the thyme when cooked
10. Take the polenta out of the fridge and cut it into 4 squares
11. Brush both sides of the polenta squares with oil and fry gently for about 10 mins
12. Add the tomatoes to the fried polenta and crumble feta on top

Potato Salad: Serves 4

Prep time/ Cook time:
5 mins / 30 mins

Ingredients:
1 tbsp olive oil

1 small onion, thinly sliced

1 garlic clove, crushed

1 tsp oregano, fresh or dried

200g cherry tomatoes

100g roasted red pepper

300g new potatoes, halved if large

25g black olives

A handful basil leaves

Method:

1. Heat the oil in a saucepan, add the onion and cook for 5-10 mins until soft

2. Add the garlic and oregano and cook for 1 min

3. Add the tomatoes and peppers, season well and simmer gently for 10 mins

4. While that's cooking, cook the potatoes in water for 10-15 mins

5. When they're cooked, mix with the sauce and serve warm, sprinkled with olives and basil

<u>Prosciutto, Fig and Mozzarella Salad: Serves 4</u>

Prep time/ Cook time:

15 mins/5 mins

Ingredients:

200g fine green beans

6 small figs, quartered

1 shallot

1 ball mozzarella

300g prosciutto

50g hazelnut, toasted and chopped

small handful of basil

3 tbsp balsamic vinegar

1 tbsp fig relish

3 tbsp olive oil

Method:

1. Cook the green beans for 2-3 mins in water until tender

2. Drain, dry and arrange on a platter

3. Add the figs, chopped shallot, mozzarella, hazelnuts and basil

4. Tear up the prosciutto and scatter over the salad

5. Mix the vinegar, fig relish, oil and seasoning and pour over the salad before serving

Halloumi and Tomato Salad with Mint: Serves 4

Prep time/ Cook time:

15 mins/5 mins

236

Ingredients:

400g chickpea

2 large tomatoes, chopped

3 spring onions, trimmed and sliced

12 leaves fresh mint, chopped

1 lemon, juiced

2 tbsp olive oil

salt and black pepper

200g halloumi cheese

Method:

1. Pop the chickpeas, tomatoes, green onions, mint, lemon juice, and olive oil in a salad bowl. Season with salt and pepper

2. Cook the halloumi in a medium hot pan for 1-2 mins per side

3. Remove from heat and chop into small chunks

4. Add to the salad and mix well. Serve warm

Desserts

Dark Chocolate Dipped Strawberries: Serves 2

Prep time/ Cook time:

5 mins

Ingredients:
1 punnet of strawberries
450g dark chocolate

Method:
1. Gently melt the dark chocolate in a bowl in the microwave, stirring at 30 second intervals
2. Hold the strawberries by the stem and dunk them into the melted chocolate
3. Let them cool and set

Chocolate Fig Balls: Serves 2

Prep time/ Cook time:
5 mins / 35 mins

Ingredients:
400g dried figs
2 tbsp almond butter
170g dark chocolate chips
2 tsp coconut oil
¾ tsp flaky sea salt

Method:
1. Line a baking sheet with baking paper
2. Combine the figs, almond butter and 2 tbsp water in a food processor

3. Blend until smooth. Use a teaspoon to measure the mixture and roll into 1 inch balls

4. Place them onto the baking sheet

5. Add the chocolate chips and oil into a bowl. Pop the bowl over a small saucepan of simmering water and stir until the chocolate is melted

6. Dip the fig balls into the chocolate to coat. Pop them back on the tray and sprinkle them with the sea salt

7. Refrigerate for 30 mins until the chocolate has set

Almond Stuffed Dates: Serves 1

Prep time/ Cook time:

5 mins

Ingredients:

4 pitted Medjool dates

4 salted whole almonds

½ tsp orange zest

Method:

1. Stuff each date with an almond and roll in orange zest

Mango Frozen Yoghurt: Serves 2

Prep time/ Cook time:

20 mins

Ingredients:

200g frozen mango chunks

5 heaped tbsp coconut yoghurt

1 lime, zested and juiced

Method:

1. Put the frozen mango, coconut yoghurt and lime juice into a blender and blitz until smooth and creamy. Sprinkle over the lime zest and serve immediately

Baked Pears: Serves 4

Prep time/ Cook time:

5 mins / 1 hour

Ingredients:

4 large pears (don't use ripe pears)

2 tbsp unsalted butter melted, plus 1 teaspoon for the pan

1 tsp pure vanilla extract

½ tsp ground cinnamon

Method:

1. Preheat your oven to 175°C

2. Butter the bottom of an edged baking dish

3. Peel and core and halve the pears, leaving the stems on. Take a slice off the bottom so that they sit upright when they cook

4. Whisk the butter, vanilla and cinnamon in a bowl

5. Brush the pears with the mixture on both sides

6. Pop the pears into the baking dish, cut side down

7. Bake for 30 mins per side, basting with the juices at intervals

Mango Parfait: Serves 2

Prep time/ Cook time:

15 mins

Ingredients:

375ml greek yoghurt

1 mango, diced

2 handfuls of pistachios

2 handfuls of pomegranate seeds

1 tsp orange blossom water

Method:

1. Mix the orange blossom water with the yoghurt and return to the fridge to chill

2. Divide the mango between two dessert bowls

3. Add some yoghurt to the bowls, covering the mango

4. Sprinkle the pistachios between the dishes

5. Top with the remaining yoghurt and decorate with pomegranate seeds

Almond Flour Cookies: Makes 10

Prep time/ Cook time:

5 mins / 16 mins

Ingredients:

112 g almond flour

3 tbsp coconut sugar

1/2 tsp baking powder

1/8 tsp fine sea salt

30ml water

Method:

1. Preheat the oven to 175°C and line a baking sheet with parchment paper
2. Whisk the almond flour, coconut sugar, baking powder and salt
3. Add the water and stir until blended
4. Drop tablespoons of the mixture on the baking sheet, spacing 2 inches apart
5. Bake for 13 to 16 minutes until golden brown and set at the centre
6. Cool for ten mins on a baking sheet before transferring to a cooling rack

Date Brownies: Makes 16

Prep time/ Cook time:

10 mins/20 mins

Ingredients:

175g pitted Medjool dates

175 ml hot water

100g almond flour

60g unsweetened cocoa powder

1/2 tsp baking powder

3 tbsp honey

2 tsp pure vanilla extract

Pinch of sea salt

Method:

1. Preheat oven to 175°C

2. Pour the hot water over the dates in a bowl and allow to sit for 10 minutes

3. Drain the water from the dates and place the dates in the bowl of a food processor or in a blender. Blitz the dates until they are smooth

4. Add the almond flour, cocoa powder, honey, vanilla and sea salt to the food processor or blender. Process again until smooth

5. Spread the mixture into an 8×8 inch pan, greased with coconut oil. Bake for 20 minutes, and allow to cool before cutting

6. Cut brownies into 16 square pieces

Apricot and Almond Pots: Serves 2

Prep time/ Cook time:

5 mins/7 mins

Ingredients:

85g dried apricots

4 tbsp apple juice

4 tbsp water

A pinch of mixed spice

6 tbsp yoghurt

1 tbsp toasted almonds

1 tsp clear honey

Method:

1. Simmer the apricots in the apple juice, water and mixed spice for 5 mins

2. Divide the mixture between 2 ramekins

3. Add the yoghurt

4. Sprinkle with almonds and honey

Olive Oil Cake: Makes 12

Prep time/ Cook time:

10 mins/50 mins

Ingredients:

4 eggs

100g granulated sweetener

110g olive oil

60g Greek yoghurt

1 tbsp lemon juice

Zest of 1 lemon

200 almond flour

30g coconut flour

½ tsp sea salt

2 tsp lemon thyme leaves

Method:

1. Preheat the oven to 180°C

2. Line an 8-inch springform tin and grease the sides

3. Whisk the eggs with an electric mixer, for 2 mins until they are frothy

4. Add the sweetener, olive oil, yoghurt, lemon juice and zest and continue mixing until well-combined

5. Stir together the almond flour, coconut flour, baking powder and salt in a separate bowl. Then add to the wet ingredients and blend until you have a smooth batter. Last, stir in the lemon thyme leaves with a spatula

6. Put the mixture into the tin and bake for 50 mins

7. Serve with Greek yoghurt

Orange, Honey and Pistachio Cake: Makes 16

Prep time/ Cook time:

15 mins/30 mins

Ingredients:

200g fine polenta

250g pistachio kernels, finely chopped

2 oranges, juiced and zested

4 eggs

175ml honey

200ml olive oil

50ml squeezed orange juice

50ml honey

Method:

1. Preheat oven to 180°C. Grease an 8inch cake tin with olive oil

2. Mix the polenta with 200g ground/chopped pistachios and orange zest from 1 of the oranges in a large bowl

3. Whisk together the eggs, 175ml honey, all the olive oil and the juice from 1 of the oranges in a large bowl

4. Pour the wet ingredients into the dry ingredients and stir together until thoroughly combined

5. Pour the batter into the tin and cook in the preheated oven for 25-30 minutes

6. Mix 50ml orange juice from the second orange with 50ml honey and pour over the hot cake whilst still in the tin

7. Leave to cook for 10 mins and then decorate with remaining pistachios and orange zest

Snacks

Roasted Chickpeas: Serves 2

Prep time/Cook time:
5 mins / 40-55 mins

Ingredients:
1 can of chickpeas, drained
1 tablespoon olive oil
1 tsp ground cumin
1 tsp chilli powder
½ tsp cayenne pepper
½ teaspoon salt

Method:
1. Preheat oven to 200°C
2. Dry the chickpeas with some kitchen rolls
3. Put the chickpeas into a bowl and add olive oil, spices and salt and mix well to coat evenly

4. Spread chickpeas out on a baking sheet lined with baking paper. Roast for 15-20 minutes

5. Mix around on a baking sheet and roast for additional 15-20 minutes, or until browned

6. Cool for 5-10 minutes and serve

Coriander, Tomato and Onion Salsa With Wholemeal Pitta: Serves 2

Prep time/Cook time:

10 mins/5 mins

Ingredients:

6 large tomatoes

Small bunch of coriander

2 wholemeal pittas

1 lime

1 small red onion

Salt and pepper

Method:

1. Half the tomatoes and discard the seeds and middle parts

2. Peel and quarter the onion

3. Strip the coriander stems and set aside the leaves

4. Squeeze the juice from the lime

5. In a food processor, blend the onion and the coriander for a few seconds until roughly chopped

6. Add the lime juice and the tomatoes and blend until it looks like salsa

7. Decant to a bowl

8. Toast the pitta

9. Season the salsa with salt and pepper and serve with the pitta

Antipasti Kebabs: Makes 6

Prep time/Cook time:
30 mins

Ingredients:
20 cherry tomatoes
20 olives, any colour
20 mini mozzarella balls
400g parma ham
2 roasted red peppers
A small bunch of basil

Method:
1. Cut in half and deseed your peppers
2. Roast them for 15-20 minutes on a medium heat until the edges are charred
3. Assemble your ingredients and some small skewers

4. Alternate your ingredients onto the skewers until you run out

5. Garnish with chopped basil

Hummus: Serves 2

Prep time/ Cook time:
10 mins

Ingredients:
400g chickpeas
juice ½ lemon
1 garlic clove
2 tbsp olive oil
2 tbsp tahini paste

Method:
1. Pop all the ingredients into a blender and pulse until smooth. Add some water to loosen if the texture is too thick

Serve with cucumber, carrot and red pepper

Salmon and Avocado Bites: Makes 12-15

Prep time/ Cook time:
10 mins

Ingredients:

1 cucumber

1 avocado

½ tbsp lime juice

170g smoked salmon

Handful of chives

Black pepper

Method:

1. Mix the lime juice and the avocado together with a fork

2. Slice the cucumber into rounds

3. Top the cucumber with the mashed avocado

4. Add salmon to each cucumber piece and sprinkle with pepper

<u>Vegetable Crisps: Serves 6</u>

Prep time/ Cook time:

15 mins/ 15 mins

Ingredients:

500g beetroot

500g sweet potatoes

400g parsnips

3 tbsp olive oil

3 lined baking sheets

Method:

1. Peel and slice the veg. Cut into thin rounds
2. Spread onto baking trays and brush with the oil, scatter sea salt on top
3. Bake for 10-12 mins until crisp

<u>Baba Ganoush Dip: Serves 6-8</u>

Prep time/ Cook time:

5 mins/25 mins

Ingredients:

3 aubergines

1-3 garlic cloves, minced

Juice of 1 lemon

2-4 tbsp tahini

3 tbsp olive oil

black pepper

1 tbsp chopped flat leaf parsley

Method:

1. Prick the aubergines with a fork
2. Grill the aubergines and turn them until the skin is charred and blacked and the flesh feels soft (about 15-20 mins)
3. Crush the garlic with the lemon juice, tahini, olive oil and pepper

4. When the aubergines have cooled, cut them in half and scoop out the flesh

5. Mix the aubergine with the garlic mix and drizzle some olive oil and parsley on top

Tomato Bruschetta: Serves 2-4

Prep time/ Cook time:

5 mins / 5 mins

Ingredients:

½ small red onion finely chopped

8 tomatoes (about 500g), coarsely chopped and drained

2-3 garlic cloves, crushed

6-8 leaves of fresh basil, finely chopped

30ml balsamic vinegar

60-80ml olive oil

1 loaf of crusty wholemeal baguette

Method:

1. Mix the onions, tomatoes, garlic and basil. Add the balsamic and the olive oil

2. Season and mix well

3. Cover and chill for an hour

4. Slice the baguette diagonally and lightly toast them

5. Spread the mixture on the warm slices of bread

Fruit and Nut bBalls: Serves 1-2

Prep time/ Cook time:

5 mins

Ingredients:

50g chopped hazelnuts

50g pecans, chopped

50g dried ready-to-eat apricots, chopped

50g Medjool dates, stones removed and chopped

2 tbsp smooth peanut butter

1 tbsp coconut oil, melted

50g desiccated coconut

1 tbsp honey

Method:

1. Pulse the pecans and hazelnuts in a food processor until fine

2. Add the apricots, dates, peanut butter, coconut oil and half the coconut to the processor and process until everything is combined

3. Add the honey and pulse again

4. Divide the mix into 14 and shape into balls

5. Spread the remaining coconut onto a plate and roll each ball in it to coat

6. Chill until firm

254

Honey Herb Walnuts: Serves 2

Prep time/ Cook time:

5 mins

Ingredients:

60g walnuts

A large sprig of rosemary

A drizzle of honey

Method:

1. Warm a pan without oil to medium heat

2. Add the walnuts and the rosemary. Stir continuously and heat until the walnuts toast

3. Remove to a plate and drizzle the honey over the top

Chapter 8

Exercising With Intermittent Fasting

This chapter is all about combining exercise with your fasting program. We'll be looking at which types of exercise are safe to do, what exercise works best with the different types of fasting, as well as things to look out for and tips to help you get the most out of combining the two.

Exercise is categorised according to intensity. High intensity, moderate and low intensity. Let's look at these below.

High intensity:

- Jogging
- Running
- HIIT- high intensity interval training
- Swimming- intense
- Cycling- hills or more than 10mph on flat terrain
- Spin classes
- Racket sports
- Heavy gardening- digging, hoeing, chopping

- Aerobics
- Circuit training

Moderate intensity exercise:

- Brisk walking
- Water aerobics
- Stair walking
- Swimming
- Weights

Low intensity exercise:

- Yoga
- Pilates
- Barre work
- Tai chi
- Gentle walking
- Stretching

So, can we safely work out while fasting? The answer in general is 'Yes', although it's a lot more nuanced than that. A lot of factors determine whether exercising is suitable for you while fasting.

- Your fitness level

- The type of fasting method that you're following
- General health
- Your diet
- The type of exercise you want to do

Before you start a fitness regime or begin exercise with fasting, it is **crucial** to talk to your doctor or a healthcare professional first.

It's important to use some common sense when it comes to exercise. If you're feeling ill or under the weather one day, then a high intensity cardio session might not be your best choice. However, a gentle Pilates session or going out for a walk in the fresh air might be more suitable.

It's necessary to listen to your body and not overdo it. Although there are studies showing that exercising with fasting has numerous benefits, we must remember that the best person to know what is right for you, is you. A good approach is to start slow. For example, it would be inadvisable to go from being a non-faster, eating three carb heavy meals a day, straight to the 'Warrior' method combining the keto diet. The same principle applies to exercise.

If you are already somebody that exercises daily and has a fairly well balanced diet, with no other health problems, then fasting and exercising together should cause you very few problems.

Let's look at some of the benefits of exercising while fasting.

Benefits of exercise when fasting

1. Potential for better fat burning

First, let's remind ourselves what happens when we fast. Our body breaks down the carbohydrates from the food that we consume and converts them to glucose. When the body doesn't need glucose for fuel, it stores it. This is called glycogen. This glycogen is released for energy when the body isn't getting food (fasting). When these stores are depleted, the body will then release fatty acids from its stores, which are taken to the liver and turned into ketones. These ketones are then used as our main energy source.

Now, our body is used to using our glycogen stores as its primary source of energy. When we exercise, the body will use those glycogen stores for energy first. However, when we are fasting and following the keto diet, our glycogen stores are already low/depleted. **(Source 1)** This means that in theory, the body will go straight to burning ketones as its energy source, therefore burning our fat stores.

2. Increases HGH levels

We know that fasting in itself, already raises the levels of HGH in our body. Exercise has also been proven to promote the production of HGH. A recent study showed that these levels are specifically higher after heavy resistance exercise, such as weight lifting. **(Source 2)**

HGH plays a massive role in body composition, cell repair and metabolism, as well as helping your body recover from injury or disease. This means the rise in HGH that you get from fasting is boosted even more by adding the element of exercise.

3. Increased motivation/ reduction in stress

When we exercise our body releases endorphins, these are 'feel-good' chemicals which make us feel happy and positive. Fasting and keto can be challenging at times. If we feel good after we exercise then that will naturally keep us motivated and excited to carry on in our fasting journey.

4. Increased Autophagy

Exercise also boosts the body's process of autophagy. Our body's cells begin a cycle of 'self cleaning'. Broken or old cells are recycled or cleared out to make way for new ones. This means that your body becomes more resilient to inflammation, protected against disease and improves our immune system.

What to look out for that might mean you need to change your routine?

- **Light-headedness**- If you're feeling light-headed or dizzy, there is a chance that the intensity of the workout is too high for you. Never push yourself beyond your reasonable limits. Also, doing fasting and exercising together can lower your blood pressure, causing light-headedness. **(Source 3)**
- **Lack of weight loss-** If you work out too intensely or over-exercise you might find that you experience a massive energy drop as well as a major rise in your appetite. As a result of this, you may end up over-eating when you get to your eating window.
- **Muscle loss-** when we enter ketosis we have burned through our glycogen stores and are now burning ketones. However, the process of ketosis doesn't always happen straight away. If we are used to primarily burning

glycogen then our body is not adapted to go straight into burning ketones for fuel instead. It might take time to become what is known as 'keto adapted'. There is a risk during this time that you may experience muscle loss. Because our body wants to hold onto the stored energy that it has for an emergency, it can sometimes begin to break down muscle instead to turn into glucose for energy. This can over time lead to muscle loss.

What kind of exercise should you do while fasting?
In general, you can do any form of exercise when fasting, as long as you are preparing your body, exercising it at the appropriate time, nourishing it and not pushing it too hard. However, there will be certain exercises that are more compatible with certain fasting methods. A lot will depend on what your body goals are with fasting. The type of exercise you should do will really depend on what your body goals are with fasting. Let's assume that if you're reading this book then your body goals are similar to what mine were. I wanted to lose the weight that had crept on since I had become perimenopausal. Gentle exercise had also given me a bit much needed head-space when I needed it. Personally, because of my endometriosis pain, I had to be careful that I didn't do anything that was too high impact that

would aggravate my pain. However, I found that low impact exercise like swimming and walking really eased my symptoms, as well as having a lovely release of endorphins that helped with my low mood.

Let's assume then that you want to exercise mainly for weight loss.

When I was growing up I remember that weight training was seen as something that beefy men in gyms did. I generally stuck to swimming and team sports, but I remember friends of mine worrying about 'bulking up'. Lifting weights isn't going to make you into the muscle man (it's not as easy as that!). Trainers and gym coaches now actually recommend weight training as the best way to lose weight. This is because, when we lift weights, your body will build muscle. Now, although this will increase your muscle mass, this doesn't mean that you won't be burning fat. Muscle tissue is more 'metabolically active' than fat tissue.

To understand this we need to understand what's called a 'basal metabolic rate'. Basically, this is the rate at which the body uses energy while completely at rest, to maintain our bodily functions, such as breathing and keeping warm. Studies have shown that after a weight training workout, our metabolism can be boosted for up to 38 hours afterwards! **(Source 4)**

This means that although you might gain some lean muscle, you'll be better off metabolically and will burn more calories.

So what about cardio? Cardio-focused work outs will not only aid weight loss but has other benefits in that it keeps your heart and lungs healthy. It also helps with sleep habits and boosts mood. A perfect workout would ideally contain elements of both cardio and weight training. So how does this fit in with fasting? Should you exercise during your fasting window or your eating window? There are some studies and professionals that say that high impact exercise is best done when you are well into your fasted state and on an empty stomach. This is to allow for maximum fat burning due to your glycogen stores being empty, or at least depleted. **(Source 5)**

Let's look at the different fasting plans and which exercises might work particularly well with each method.

Beginner level faster: 12:12 method, spontaneous fasting, the 14/10 method
For the first few weeks of beginning your fasting plan, it's probably best to get into the swing of the food plan before you tackle exercise. During this time it's possible

that you might have keto flu while your body becomes 'keto adapted'.

While your body is at this stage and potentially not in ketosis yet, it's better to do low intensity exercise. Shorter workouts and workouts from the low and moderate impact lists are best. While you are building up to longer fasting windows by following one of the beginner level fasting plans, low impact workouts such as yoga and pilates are perfect exercises to do during your eating window, or during your fasting window.

Intermediate level faster: 16/8 method, 5:2, crescendo method

As we know, the 5:2 diet has two days out of seven when your calories are super low, coming in between 500-600 a day. On these days it's best to stick to low intensity exercise and leave your high intensity exercise for the days when you are eating normally.

With the 16/8 plan, a lot of people schedule their eating window to fall between 10 am and 6 pm. This way you can benefit from having a late breakfast, a small lunch and an evening meal before your fasting window reopen. There are studies to suggest that following the 16/8 fasting method as well as exercising before your fasting window ends, can be extra beneficial to weight loss. **(Source 6)**

Advanced level: alternate day/eat stop eat

As with the 5:2 diet, it's recommended that you save your high intensity workouts for days that you aren't fasting. However, this will depend on how well adapted your body is to fasting. If you're used to exercising on an empty stomach, then there's no reason not to continue. Just remember to listen to your body.

Expert Level: warrior diet

The founder of the warrior diet recommends a mixture of high intensity and low intensity exercise, to be performed during your fasting window. However, I would be very cautious about doing anything too strenuous, due to the side effects of this particular plan. Dizziness and fatigue are rife with this method and for me, the thought of adding high intensity exercise seems like a risk. Before beginning any elements of the warrior plan, it is essential to talk it through with a doctor or healthcare provider. I would recommend if you do try the warrior method, that you stick to very low intensity exercise, such as swimming or walking.

Tips on how to exercise while intermittent fasting

- Ease into it!- as I've said before about fasting, this is a marathon, not a sprint. Your fitness journey, like your fasting journey, is a personal thing, dependent on many factors.

If you aren't used to exercising, then build your workouts slowly as your body adjusts, not only to exercise but fasting.

- Think about your schedule- make a plan that revolves around your lifestyle. For example, if you know that you are more suited to morning exercise, then schedule your exercise for that time. Perhaps you work shifts? Or nights? Plan your eating window and your exercise accordingly.

- Hydrate, hydrate, hydrate- it's imperative to keep hydrated when we fast, but it's even more crucial when you combine that with exercise too. When you fast, you lose on average 20% of the water that your body would normally get from food. Now add exercise and the water that you lose from sweating and you've got even more reason to keep hydrated.

- Don't overdo it- at the end of the day, this whole process should be about being healthy. While it's good to challenge ourselves and push to attain our goals, there's no sense in burning yourself out in the process. There will be days when you have more energy than others. It's important to listen to your body and honour its needs.

- Variety- if possible, try different types of exercise with varying intensity into your daily routine. Keep your body alert by alternating cardio with yoga or Pilates, or throw in a weights session.

- Flexibility- be open to changing up exercise plans if they aren't working for you, or fitting in with your life. Sometimes it takes a while to get a fasting and exercise plan that works for you. Maybe your fasting window is too long? Or you've discovered that you really can't forgo breakfast so you need to change the times of your fasting window so you can work out in the evening instead? There's no shame in adjusting or changing something to work for you and your needs.

Chapter 9
Frequently Asked Questions

This chapter looks at some frequently asked questions that many people have when they are embarking on an intermittent fasting/keto plan.

1. Why am I not losing weight?
- You might be eating too many calories – tracking your calories can be helpful in identifying any patterns in your eating habits. It's easy to overeat when you're feeling hungry from fasting. Downloading a calorie counting app might be a good way of tracking exactly what you're eating and when.
- Lack of ketosis- if you're following the keto diet with your fasting plan, it's likely that your body will regularly be entering ketosis. However, it's not a given. You can buy different types of keto monitors, such as breath tests or urine strips. This might give you an idea of what your body is up to, you can then tweak your diet accordingly.
- You aren't eating well- not all calories are created equally. If you find that your diet mainly consists of fast food (even if it's keto) you are less likely to lose weight. Try to plan your menus

around nutrient-dense foods that fill you up for longer.

- Don't always go by the scale- Sometimes we lose inches rather than weight, taking your measurements at the beginning of your journey will help you more accurately measure your progress, especially if you're feeling defeated if the scales aren't moving

2. How do you combat hunger pains?

- Keep hydrated- sometimes the body confuses thirst with hunger. Make sure that you drink an adequate amount of liquid to rule out the possibility that you are dehydrated.
- Hot drinks- in addition to keeping you hydrated, a warm keto friendly hot drink such as black coffee or a tasty herbal tea can really take the edge off hunger pangs.
- Sleep- scheduling your fasting windows so that a big chunk of it falls when you are asleep is a good way to avoid hunger pangs. When I was doing the 5:2 diet I would usually head to bed as early as possible to avoid the dreaded evening munchies.
- Distract yourself- hunger is often mistaken for boredom. Many people have got into the habit of eating for the sake of eating. Learning to

differentiate between true hunger and fancying food, is a process. While you figure this out, the distraction technique is a good way of avoiding hunger pangs. Take a bath, sort out a drawer or do some exercise. Your eating window will roll around before you know it.

3. How do I prevent constipation?

- Eat enough fibre- fibre keeps our digestive system happy and our stools soft, and it also promotes good gut health.
- Stay hydrated- Try to aim for 6-8 glasses of water a day, to prevent constipation.
- Exercise- exercises based on stretching and muscle work can help to keep our body from getting constipated. Yoga is particularly good for relieving the pressure of constipation.

4. What can I do to help the symptoms of keto flu?

- Stay hydrated- I know I keep saying it, but keeping hydrated really will help. When we follow a keto diet we lose a lot of our water stores. Keep yourself nicely hydrated to prevent dehydration.
- Take it easy- don't do anything too strenuous for the first few weeks of your keto diet. Your body is getting used to a whole new fuel source. Don't

stress it out or embark on an intensive new exercise regime.

- Keep your electrolyte levels up- our kidneys release sodium from the body when our insulin levels decrease. Making sure that we have enough salt is important. **(Source 1)**
- Ensure you're getting nutrients- the restrictive nature of the keto diet means that it's easy to miss out on certain nutrients, especially at the beginning when you are getting used to the plan. For example, potassium-rich foods are limited to keto (bananas, beans and starchy vegetables) Make sure you eat keto friendly foods that are rich in nutrients you might miss out on. Another nutrient that might help with symptoms of keto flu, is magnesium. Magnesium helps with headaches and is good for regulating sleep. **(Source 2)**
- Sleep- Keeping your body well rested is so important. Keto flu can be made worse when your body is sleep deprived as the body releases the stress hormone cortisol. This in turn makes symptoms of keto flu even worse. **(Source 3)**

5. Can you do keto with plant based protein sources?
Yes, you can. Many plant based proteins such as tofu, nuts, leafy green vegetables and seeds are compatible with the keto diet. However, keto will be more

restrictive if you are vegan and completely plant based. If you are looking to cut *down* on your animal protein consumption for ethical or environmental reasons, but still eat eggs and dairy, then it will be easier. There are people that follow a vegan keto diet, but their diet is extremely restrictive and there is a greater risk of malnutrition and potential for illness due to lack of nutrients.

Having said that, there is nothing wrong with enjoying the variety of keto friendly vegetables, seeds and nuts that make up a big part of the plant-based diet. In my opinion, though, it's probably best to not have restriction of the vegan plan on top of the keto and instead to be able to have some flexibility with your food choices.

6. What are these abbreviations?
- OMAD- one meal a day – usually in the context of a fasting plan with a small eating window like the Warrior method, or spontaneous meal skipping
- ADF- Alternate day fasting
- IF- intermittent fasting
- NSV- non-scale victory – usually in reference to a positive occurrence as a result of the plan, that isn't to do with weight loss.

- LCHF/HFLC- low carb high fat or high fat low carb
- BF- body fat
- HGH- human growth hormone
- ACV- Apple cider vinegar

7. Which are the best supplements to take?

As always, this is just a general guide and before taking any supplements you should ALWAYS check with your healthcare provider.

- As the keto diet restricts certain foods, it's important to make sure that we make good choices and get the full range of nutrients from the keto foods that we do eat. However, this isn't always possible. Taking a supplement can help with this.
- Magnesium- this nutrient supports good sleep, our immune system and regulates our blood sugar levels. Many magnesium-rich foods are high in carbs and off-limits on the keto plan.
- Potassium- potassium is essential for nerve and cell function as well as being essential for brain health. As with magnesium, potassium-rich foods are also limited on keto, with the majority of potassium coming from beans and legumes.

274

Avocados, are a rich source of potassium however and can be enjoyed freely on keto.

- Omega 3- a lack of omega 3 can cause inflammation in our body. This is particularly important to avoid in our menopause, as our bodies are already prone to inflammation. Omega 3 is present in oily fish, however, not everyone eats enough of it to combat any imbalance. Taking a supplement can be useful in correcting that. **(Source 4)**

- Vitamin B- B vitamins help to prevent strokes, heart disease and dementia. B-6 and B-12 vitamins can help to support cognitive function and B-6 can even help with the symptoms of depression in women. B-9 has also been found to be effective in reducing the amount of hot flashes you might experience

- Vitamin D- most people are deficient in Vitamin D (unless you live in a very sunny climate!) Vitamin D is essential for bone health, which is particularly important to menopausal women, due to our increased risk of osteoporosis.

- Passiflora/ Passionflower- can help with the symptoms of anxiety as well as sleep problems, muscle cramps and other symptoms associated with menopause.

Sources

Chapter 1

1. https://www.engage.england.nhs.uk/safety-and-innovation/menopause-in-the-workplace
2. https://www.endocrine.org/patient-engagement/endocrine-library/menopause
3. How Menopause Affects Your Immune System - Renew Youth
4. Menopause and heart and circulatory conditions | BHF
5. Fasting: the history , pathophysiology and complications - PubMed (nih.gov)

Chapter 2

1. Changes in hunger and fullness in relation to gut peptides before and after 8 weeks of alternate day fasting - PubMed (nih.gov)
2. Randomized cross-over trial of short-term water-only fasting: metabolic and cardiovascular consequences - PubMed (nih.gov)

2.A Fasting: the history, pathophysiology and complications - PubMed (nih.gov)

3. The effect of fasting or calorie restriction on autophagy induction: A review of the literature – ScienceDirect

4. INTERMITTENT FASTING AND HUMAN METABOLIC HEALTH – PMC (nih.gov)

5. Glucose tolerance and skeletal muscle gene expression in response to alternate day fasting - PubMed (nih.gov)

6. The effects of intermittent or continuous energy restriction on weight loss and metabolic disease risk markers: a randomized trial in young overweight women - PubMed (nih.gov)

7. Intermittent Fasting For Women - Dr. Jolene Brighten (drbrighten.com)

8. Targeting Autophagy in Cancer: Recent Advances and Future Directions | Cancer Discovery | American Association for Cancer Research (aacrjournals.org)

9. Short-term fasting induces profound neuronal autophagy - PubMed (nih.gov)

10. Intermittent fasting interventions for treatment of overweight and obesity in adults: a systematic review and meta-analysis - PubMed (nih.gov) Dietary Intake Regulates the Circulating Inflammatory Monocyte Pool: Cell

11. Dietary Intake Regulates the Circulating Inflammatory Monocyte Pool: Cell

12. Safety, health improvement and well-being during a 4 to 21-day fasting period in an observational study including 1422 subjects - PubMed (nih.gov)

Chapter 4

1. New Insight into Diabetes Management: From Glycemic Index to Dietary Insulin Index - PubMed (nih.gov) Ghrelin – Physiological Functions and Regulation - PMC (nih.gov)

   1.1Physiology, Leptin - StatPearls - NCBI Bookshelf (nih.gov)

2. Flipping the Metabolic Switch: Understanding and Applying Health Benefits of Fasting - PMC (nih.gov)
3. Intermittent fasting vs daily calorie restriction for type 2 diabetes prevention: a review of human findings - ScienceDirect
4. Nutritional Ketosis with Ketogenic Diets or Exogenous Ketones: Features, Convergence, and Divergence - PubMed (nih.gov)
5. Ketosis, ketogenic diet and food intake control: a complex relationship – PMC (nih.gov)
6. Neuroprotective and disease-modifying effects of the ketogenic diet – PMC (nih.gov)

7. Effects of beta-hydroxybutyrate on cognition in memory-impaired adults -PubMed (nih.gov)

8. Role for brain-derived neurotrophic factor in learning and memory – PubMed (nih.gov) Full article: Short-term fasting induces profound neuronal autophagy (tandfonline.com)

9. Therapeutic targeting of autophagy in neurodegenerative and infectious diseases - PMC (nih.gov)

10. Autophagy in health and disease: A comprehensive review - PubMed (nih.gov)

11. Intermittent fasting vs daily calorie restriction for type 2 diabetes prevention: a review of human findings - PubMed (nih.gov)

12. Augmented growth hormone (GH) secretory burst frequency and amplitude mediate enhanced GH secretion during a two-day fast in normal men | The Journal of Clinical Endocrinology & Metabolism | Oxford Academic (oup.com)

13. Prolonged fasting reduces IGF-1/PKA to promote hematopoietic-stem-cell-based regeneration and reverse immunosuppression - PubMed (nih.gov)

14. Fasting and cancer: molecular mechanisms and clinical application – PMC (nih.gov)

Chapter 5

1. Evaluating the Patient With Diarrhea: A Case-Based Approach - PMC (nih.gov)
2. Time-restricted feeding plus resistance training in active females: a randomized trial | The American Journal of Clinical Nutrition | Oxford Academic (oup.com)
3. Nature and Science of Sleep | Aims and Scope - Dove Press Open Access Publisher
4. High Protein Intake Stimulates Postprandial GLP1 and PYY Release – PMC (nih.gov)

5. Fasting as a Therapy in Neurological Disease - PMC (nih.gov)
6. Ketogenic Diet - StatPearls - NCBI Bookshelf (nih.gov)
7. Hypothalamic mTOR signaling regulates food intake - PubMed (nih.gov)

Chapter 6

1. Caffeine intake increases plasma ketones: an acute metabolic study in humans -PubMed (nih.gov)
2. The effects of high protein diets on thermogenesis, satiety and weight loss: a critical review - PubMed (nih.gov)

3. Effect of Dietary Protein on Bone Loss in Elderly Men and Women: The Framingham Osteoporosis Study - Hannan - 2000 - Journal of Bone and Mineral Research - Wiley Online Library

4. Fish consumption, omega-3 fatty acids and risk of heart failure: a meta-analysis- PubMed (nih.gov)

5. Fish consumption and cognitive decline with age in a large community study -PubMed (nih.gov)

6. Omega-3 fatty acids and blood pressure - PubMed (nih.gov)

7. Vitamins and minerals - Vitamin C - NHS (www.nhs.uk)

7a. Monounsaturated Fat | American Heart Association

7b. Saturated Fats and Health: A Reassessment and Proposal for Food-Based Recommendations: JACC State-of-the-Art Review - ScienceDirect

7c. Facts about polyunsaturated fats: MedlinePlus Medical Encyclopedia

8. Intermittent fasting during Ramadan attenuates proinflammatory cytokines and immune cells in healthy subjects – PubMed (nih.gov)

9. The effect of prolonged fasting on levels of growth hormone-binding protein and free growth hormone - PubMed (nih.gov)

10. Intermittent fasting vs daily calorie restriction for type 2 diabetes prevention: a review of human findings - PubMed (nih.gov)

11. The Effects of a Low-Carbohydrate Ketogenic Diet and a Low-Fat Diet on Mood, Hunger, and Other Self-Reported Symptoms - McClernon - 2007 - Obesity – Wiley Online Library

12. Insulin resistance, obesity, hypertension, and renal sodium transport -PubMed (nih.gov)

13. Low-carbohydrate diets: nutritional and physiological aspects – PubMed (nih.gov)

14. Mediterranean Diet Effects on Type 2 Diabetes Prevention, Disease Progression, and Related Mechanisms. A Review - PMC (nih.gov)

15. The Mediterranean Diet and Cardiovascular Health - PubMed (nih.gov)

Chapter 7

Keto breakfasts

1. Recipe: Crispy Keto Breakfast Cereal – KETO- MOJO RecipeEric Lundy

282

Keto dinners

1. Keto Lemon-Garlic Chicken Thighs in the Air Fryer Recipe (allrecipes.com)
2. Gordon Ramsay butter chicken | Indian Recipes | GoodTo
3. Keto Zucchini Lasagna - (Gluten Free) Recipe - Diet Doctor

Keto sides

1. Easy Keto Coleslaw Recipe With Creamy Low-Carb Dressing - by My Keto Kitchen
2. Garlic Parmesan Roasted Asparagus - Belle of the Kitchen

Keto snacks

1. Low-Carb Kale Chips – Vegan Snack Recipe – Diet Doctor

Keto desserts

1. Top Keto Dessert Recipes - Diet Doctor
2. Keto Lemon Bars - Hey Keto Mama

Mediterranean breakfasts

1. Shakshuka With Feta Recipe - NYT Cooking (nytimes.com)

2. Tropical Overnight Oats Recipe | EatingWell
3. Sweet Potato Hash with Eggs - Mediterranean Living
4. Parmesan Spinach Cakes Recipe | EatingWell

Mediterranean lunches

1. Bulgur wheat salad | Sainsbury`s Magazine (sainsburysmagazine.co.uk)
2. Fig & Goat Cheese Salad Recipe | EatingWell
3. Greek Lemon Chicken Soup - Damn Delicious
4. Spaghetti alle vongole recipe | BBC Good Food
5. Chicken Quinoa Bowl - The Harvest Kitchen
6. Harissa Chickpea Stew with Eggplant and Millet (purewow.com)

Mediterranean dinners

1. Mediterranean Fish Stew (30 minute recipe) - Mediterranean Living
2. Moroccan chicken with chickpeas | Tesco Real Food
3. Lamb Stew With Spinach & Garbanzos - Mediterranean Living
4. Prawns with new potatoes and peas – One pot wonders Lindsey Bareham
5. Mediterranean Baked Cod - Mediterranean Living

6. Mediterranean salmon recipe | delicious. magazine (deliciousmagazine.co.uk)
7. Seafood Paella Recipe | Rice Recipes | Tesco Real Food
8. Chicken Breast Stuffed with Feta & Roasted Red Pepper Recipe | EatingWell
9. Ricotta, broccoli & lemon penne recipe | BBC Good Food
10. Pork Stifado One pot wonders, Lindsey Bareham
11. Simple Oven-Baked Sea Bass Recipe - Food.com

Mediterranean snacks

1. Spicy Roasted Chickpeas Recipe by Tasty
2. Mediterranean Antipasto Skewers - A Cedar Spoon
3. Smoked Salmon, Avocado and Cucumber Bites - Downshiftology
4. Vegetable crisps | British Recipes | GoodTo
5. Vegetable crisps | British Recipes | GoodTo
6. Baba ganoush recipe - BBC Food
7. Fruit and Nut Energy Balls - Recipes - RH Uncovered
8. Tomato bruschetta recipe | BBC Good Food

Mediterranean sides

1. Greek Spinach and Rice recipe (Spanakorizo) - My Greek Dish
2. Tricolore couscous salad recipe | BBC Good Food
3. Lemony Asparagus With Garlic - Mediterranean Living
4. Crisp Polenta with Roasted Cherry Tomatoes Recipe - Cook.me Recipes
5. Mediterranean potato salad recipe | BBC Good Food
6. Mediterranean fig & mozzarella salad recipe | BBC Good Food
7. Halloumi, Chickpea, and Tomato Salad with Mint (allrecipes.com)

Mediterranean dessert ideas

1. Chocolate Fig Bites - Fully Mediterranean
2. Mango Froyo Recipe | olivemagazine
3. No-Sugar-Added Baked Pears - Healthy Recipes Blog (healthyrecipesblogs.com)
4. Mediterranean Parfait (honestcooking.com)
5. 3-Ingredient Almond Flour Cookies {V, GF, oil-free) | powerhungry®
6. How To Make Fudgy Gluten-Free Brownies With Dates (mindbodygreen.com)

7. Warm apricot & almond pots recipe | BBC Good Food

8. Keto Almond Flour Olive Oil Cake – Sugar Free Londoner

9. Orange, Pistachio and Honey Polenta Cake - Easy Peasy Foodie

Chapter 8

1. Exercising in the Fasted State Reduced 24-Hour Energy Intake in Active Male Adults - PMC (nih.gov)

2. Acute resistance exercise stimulates sex-specific dimeric immunoreactive growth hormone responses – ScienceDirect

3. Intermittent Fasting in Cardiovascular Disorders—An Overview – PMC (nih.gov)

4. Effect of an acute period of resistance exercise on excess post-exercise oxygen consumption: implications for body mass management

5. SpringerLinkExercising in the Fasted State Reduced 24-Hour Energy Intake in Active Male Adults - PMC (nih.gov)

6. Effects of eight weeks of time-restricted feeding (16/8) on basal metabolism, maximal strength, body composition, inflammation, and cardiovascular risk factors in resistance-trained

males | Journal of Translational Medicine | Full Text (biomedcentral.com)

Chapter 9

1. Insulin resistance, obesity, hypertension, and renal sodium transport - PubMed (nih.gov)
2. Magnesium in Prevention and Therapy - PMC (nih.gov)
3. Effects of sleep deprivation on serum cortisol level and mental health in servicemen - PubMed (nih.gov)
4. Health Implications of High Dietary Omega-6 Polyunsaturated Fatty Acids -PMC (nih.gov)